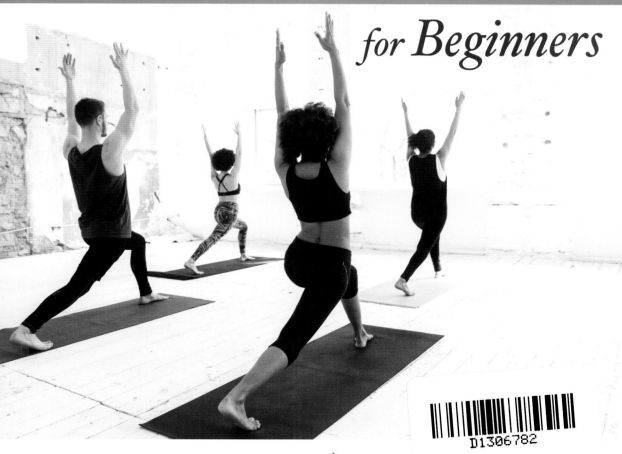

YOGA

for Beginners

Publications International, Ltd.

Consultant: Barb Sheridan

Model: Meghan Khanna

Photography: Christopher Hiltz

Additional images from Shutterstock.com

ISBN: 978-1-64030-875-6

Manufactured in China.

8 7 6 5 4 3 2 1

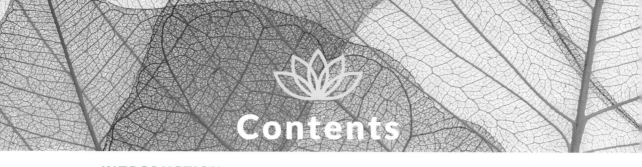

Contents

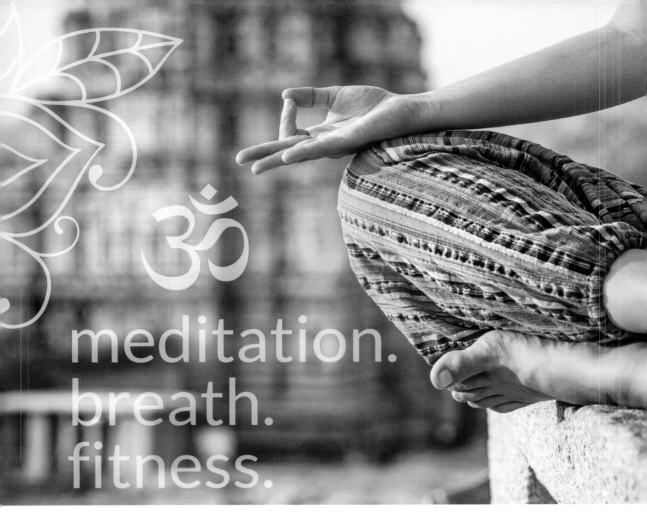

meditation.
breath.
fitness.

Yoga Is for Everyone

What we think of today as just "yoga" is a modern and adapted form of an ancient spiritual practice from Hinduism. Modern westernized yoga is one part meditation, one part breath awareness, and one part fitness.

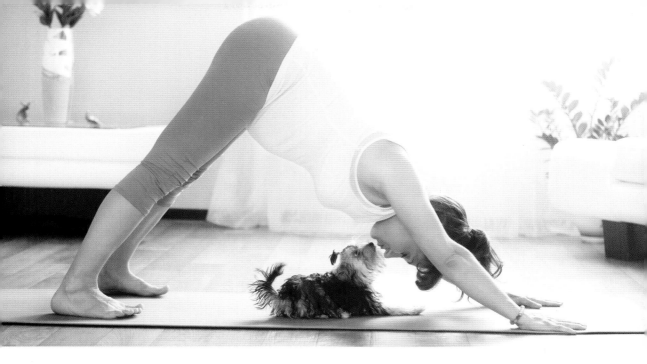

As yoga entered the western mainstream beginning as early as the 1920s, people quickly realized how effective these stretches and strength exercises were, with the added benefit of relaxing and meditative breathing. Yoga is for everyone: all ability levels can begin with sitting and breathing, no special equipment or clothes or classes required. There are also support pieces—like blocks, blankets, and straps—to make yoga doable for more people.

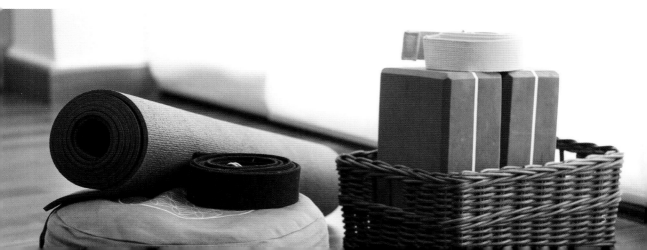

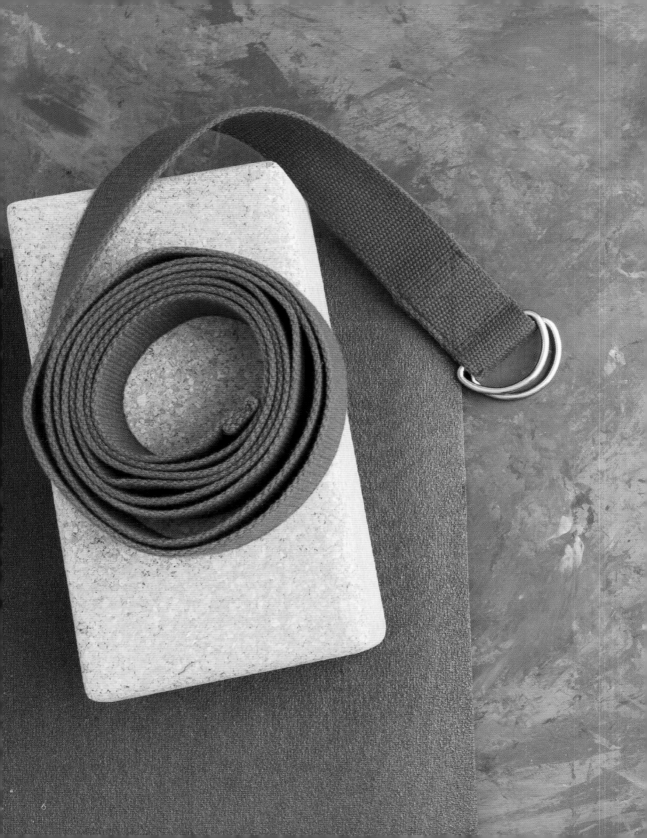

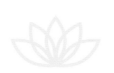

Yoga Blocks

Yoga blocks are sturdy foam supports that you can lean on or use to support your body as you practice poses. Throughout the book, you'll find cues for when to use blocks if you need them, and photos of those blocks in use. But they're really for you to use whenever you want added stability.

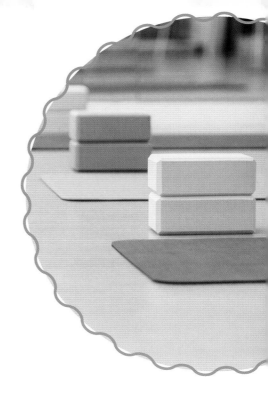

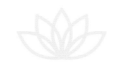

Straps

A strap can help you with poses that require you to reach your toes, for example—removing an obstacle for those who can't reach their toes, have joint problems, or any other reason. You can buy straps at yoga or sporting goods stores, but you can also use a jump rope, a woven scarf, or even a length of rope or canvas webbing from the hardware store.

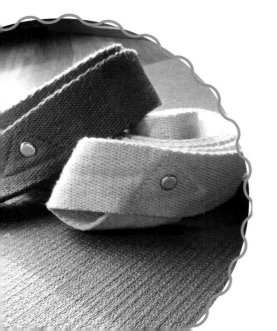

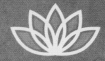

Bolsters & Blankets

A regular woven blanket makes a great support item for yoga practice. Fold the blanket into a comfortable bolster shape and use it anytime you need more cushion. Blankets are especially good for keeping your knees supported and engaged so you don't lock them in place.

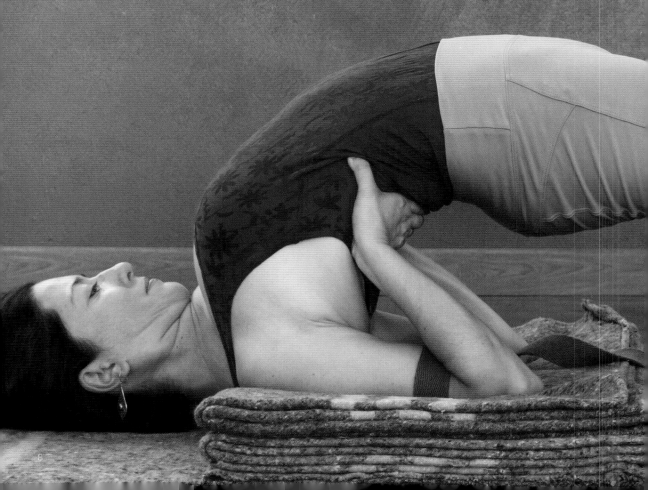

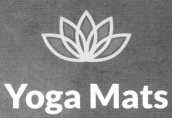

Yoga Mats

The quintessential yoga equipment is the mat, which is a thin, tough, and soft piece of foam rubber. There are cheap yoga mats available almost everywhere, giving you a great way to try yoga without needing to invest in a quality mat first.

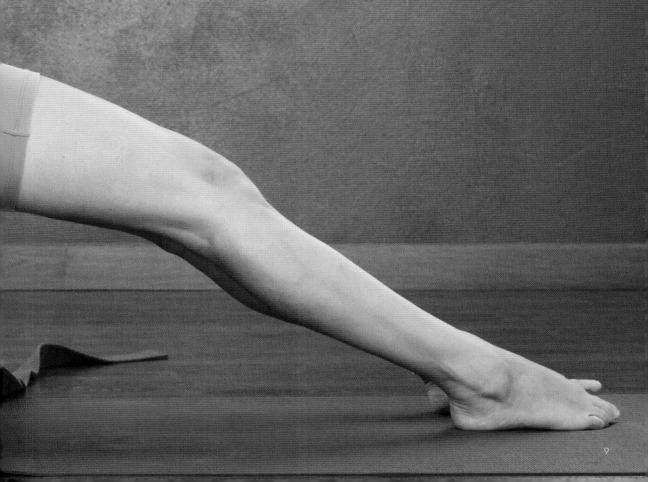

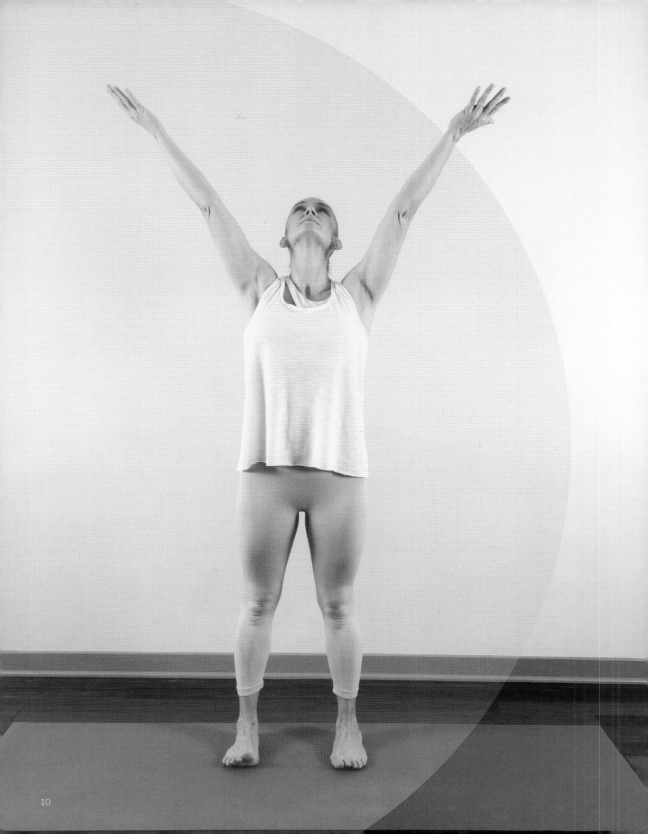

Standing Poses

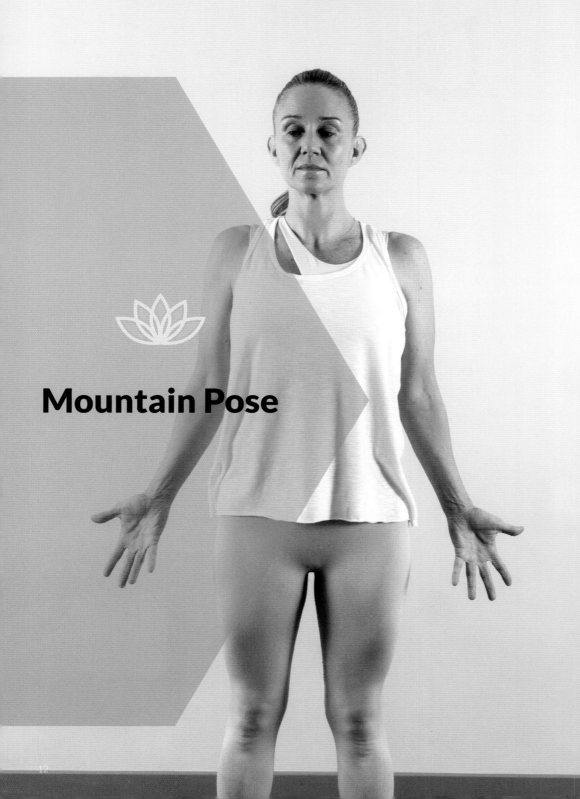

Mountain Pose

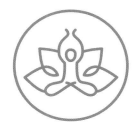

Mountain pose is a simple and centering pose. Stand with your feet about hips width apart, parallel to each other. Ground through your feet and relax your toes. Line your shoulders up directly over your hips and draw your shoulder blades toward each other behind your back. Turn your palms forward and actively spread your fingers. Feel the top of your head reach toward the ceiling as you elongate your spine. Whether your toes are gently resting or lifting up, feel the ball of your foot and your heel forming a steady base. Breathe gently in and out your nose.

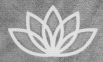

Upward Salute

Upward salute pose is a good one to follow mountain pose. Keep your feet parallel and hips width apart, with toes relaxed. Raise your arms over your head, with palms facing each other. You can spread your fingers out or hold them loosely together. Feel the stretch in your back and sides. Let your shoulders drop as

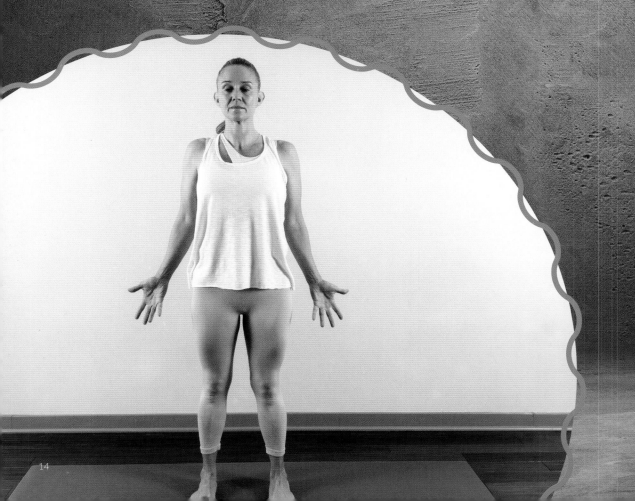

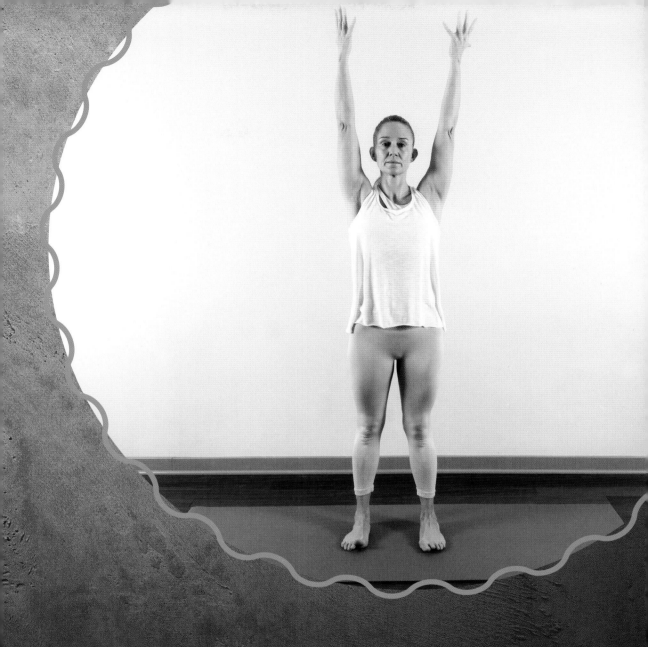

you lengthen and relax your neck. Work toward bringing your straight arms back behind your ears. Feel the sensation of your whole body lengthening, from your fingertips all the way down to your grounded feet.

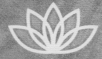

Standing Forward Fold

Standing forward fold pose is a forward stretch that can meet any level of flexibility. Stand with feet hips width apart and parallel. Keep your knees gently bent instead of locked straight. Hinge from your hips and fold forward toward the floor. If your fingers don't touch the floor, rest your hands on a set of yoga

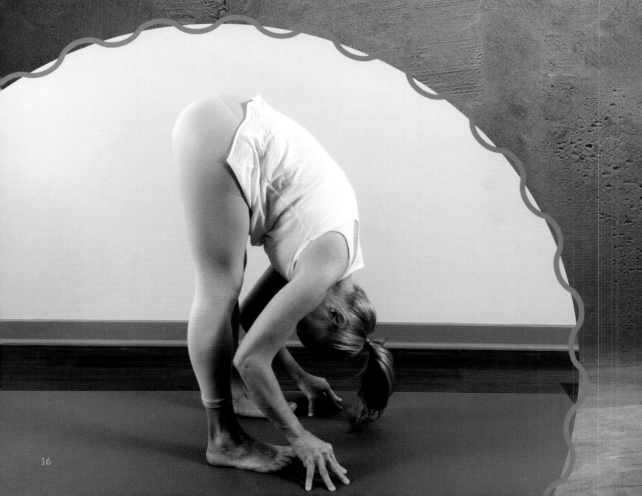

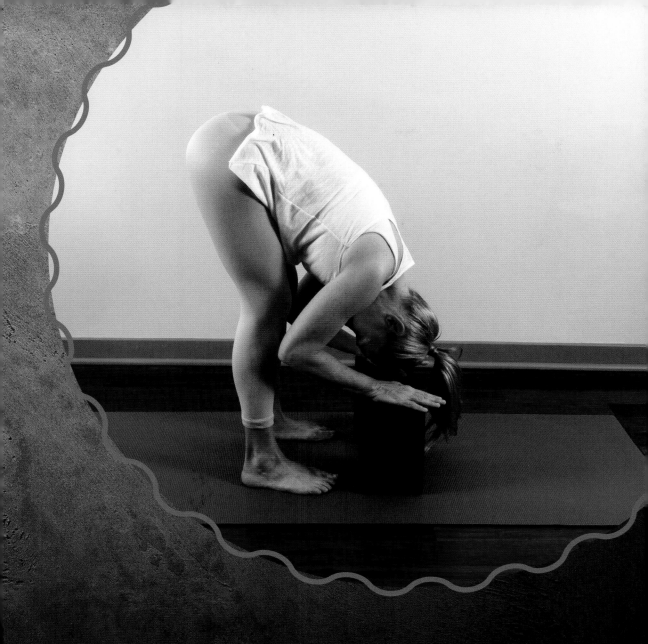

blocks as pictured above. Using
yoga blocks is a great way to feel
comfortable and be confident
doing stretches—in this case, you
can rest your hands on the blocks
and let your arms relax as you feel
the stretch in your back and legs.
Keep your hips aligned over your
ankles and let your neck relax as
your back lengthens.

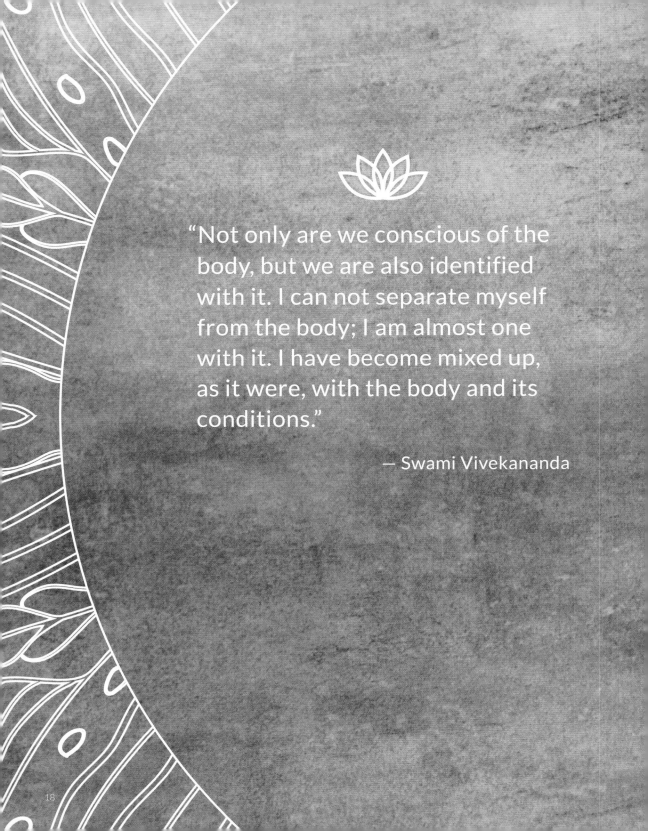

"Not only are we conscious of the body, but we are also identified with it. I can not separate myself from the body; I am almost one with it. I have become mixed up, as it were, with the body and its conditions."

— Swami Vivekananda

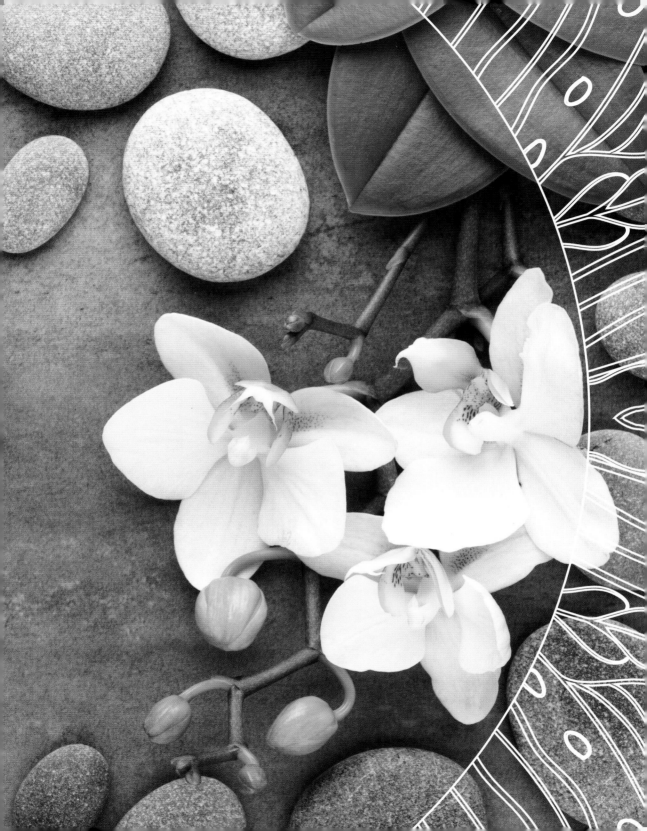

Half Standing
Forward Fold

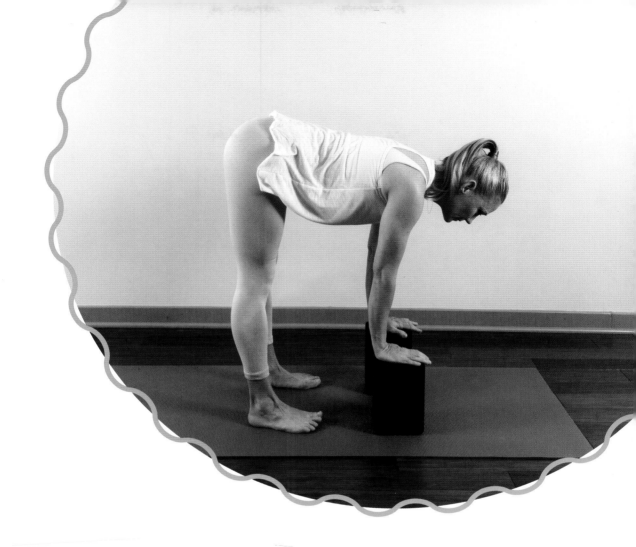

Half standing forward fold pose is a great addition or alternative to standing forward fold pose. This pose creates a slightly different stretch and sensation in your body. With feet hips width apart and parallel, hinge at your hips and rest your hands flat against your shins, your thighs, or on yoga blocks as pictured here. Keep your back flat. It's okay to bend your arms as they rest on the blocks so that your back forms a 90° angle to your legs. Feel your chest reaching forward and let your jaw soften and relax as you also soften your breath.

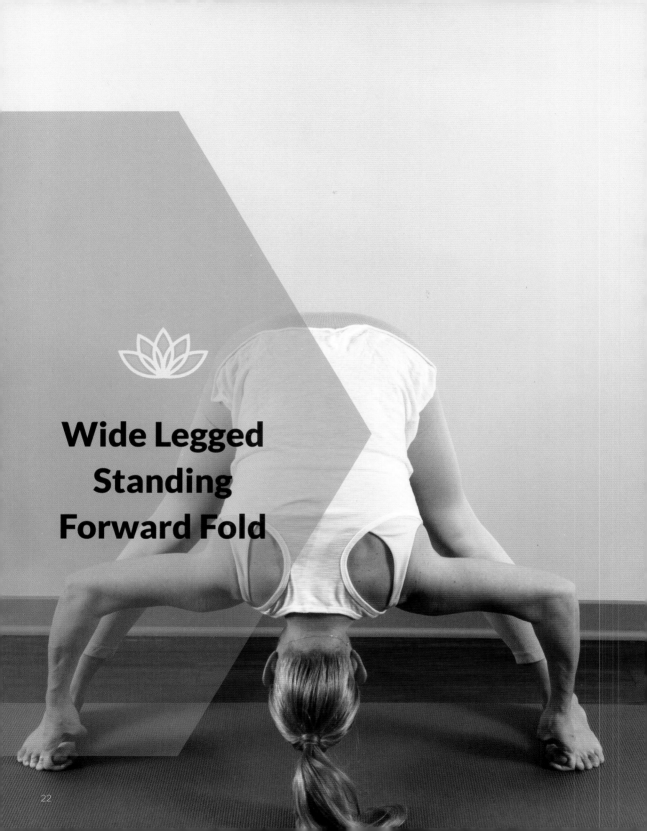

Wide Legged
Standing
Forward Fold

Wide legged standing forward fold pose is still a forward stretch but with the added difference of a wide stance. If using yoga blocks, keep them in place from the previous pose.

Walk your legs apart with your toes pointing in slightly and your heels angled out. Place your hands on your outer shins, the floor, or rest them flat on blocks as pictured on page 24.

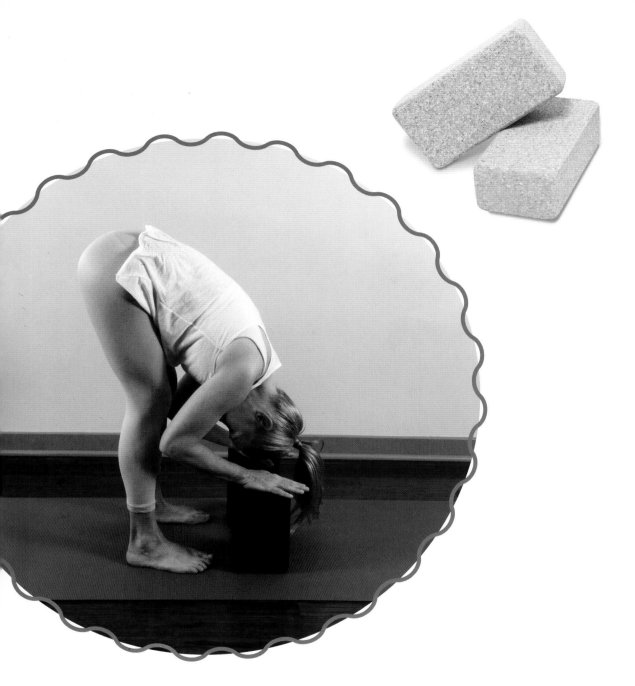

Keep your hips in line with your ankles as you fold. Feel the stretch in your back and legs, but avoid hyper-extending your knees. Let your neck relax as you stretch. Feel your back lengthen as you breathe in and out.

If you wish to take wide legged standing forward fold into a deeper variation, you can hold onto your ankles, your outer feet or wrap your two "peace fingers" and thumbs around your big toes. This will create a "bind" to allow you to fold more deeply into the pose. Continue to lengthen as you breathe in and out of your nose.

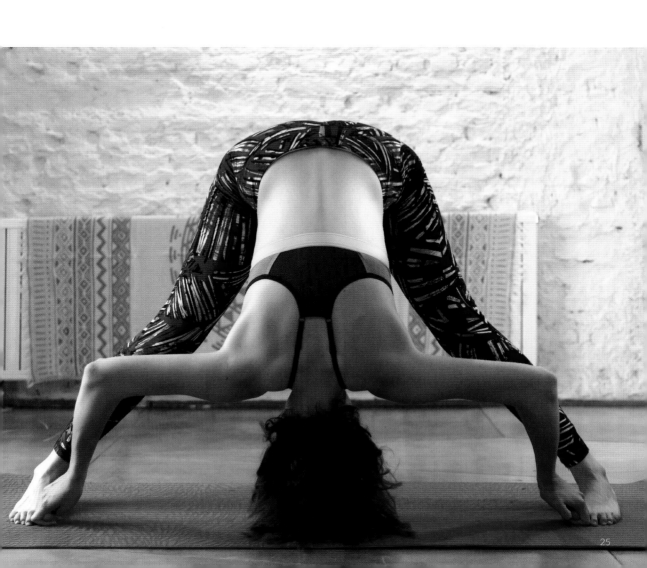

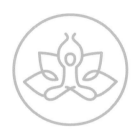

Revolved Wide-Legged Standing Forward Fold

This is a forward stretch and mild balance exercise. Start in a wide-legged standing forward fold, with your hands on the mat or blocks directly below your shoulders. Keep your hips even as you lift one hand and move it in a smooth arc toward the ceiling. Rotate your shoulders and turn your head to gaze upward as you extend your hand to the ceiling.

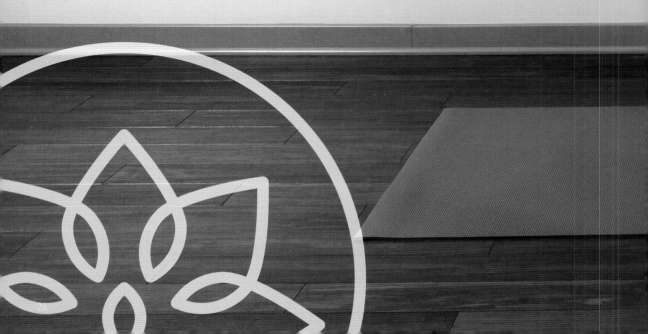

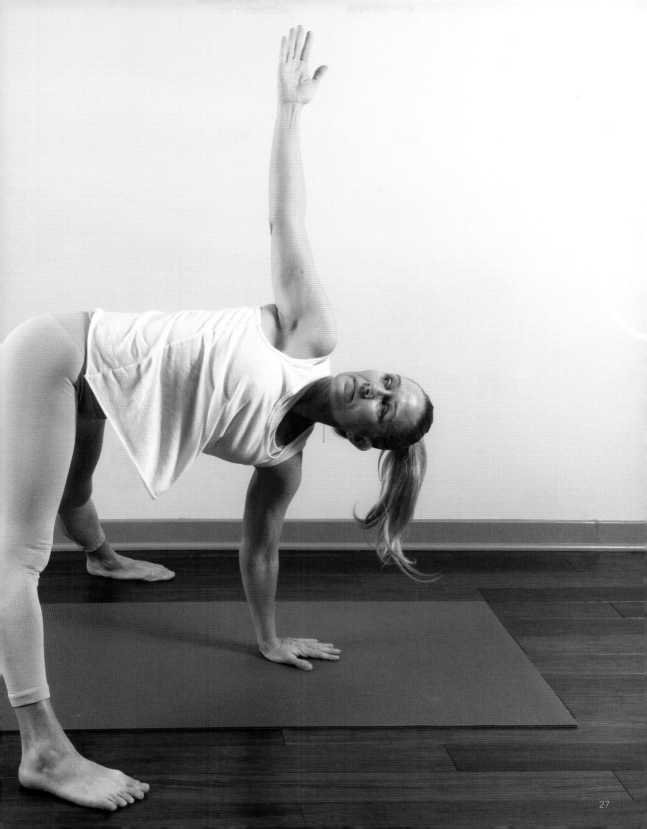

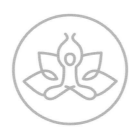

Revolved Wide-Legged Standing Forward Fold

Because of the balance and twisting, this pose can be tricky. Use a block beneath your bottom hand to help stabilize you, if needed. You can also keep your top arm bent with your hand resting on your hip or lower back, twisting gently as far as is comfortable.

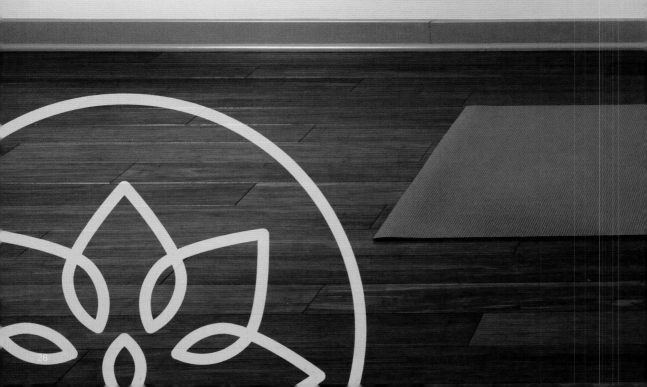

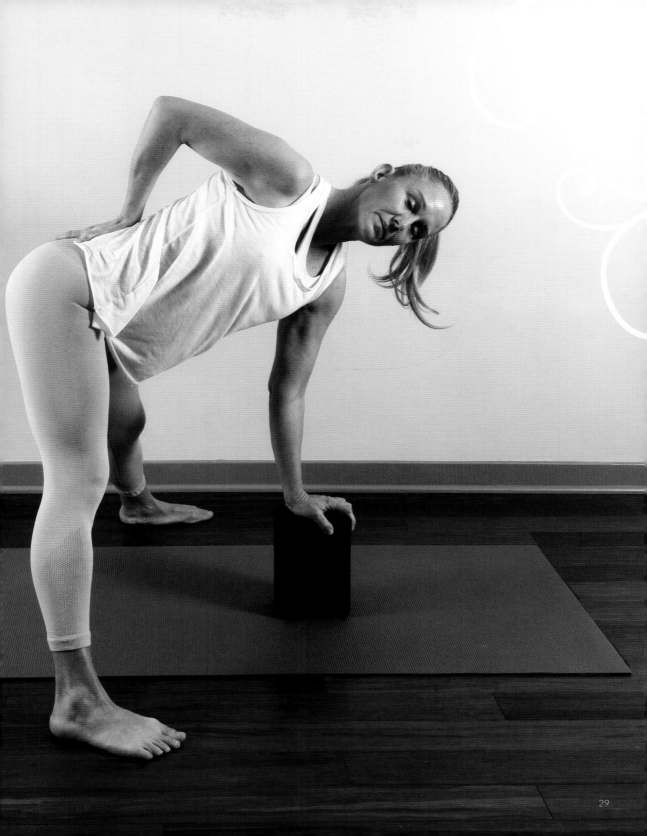

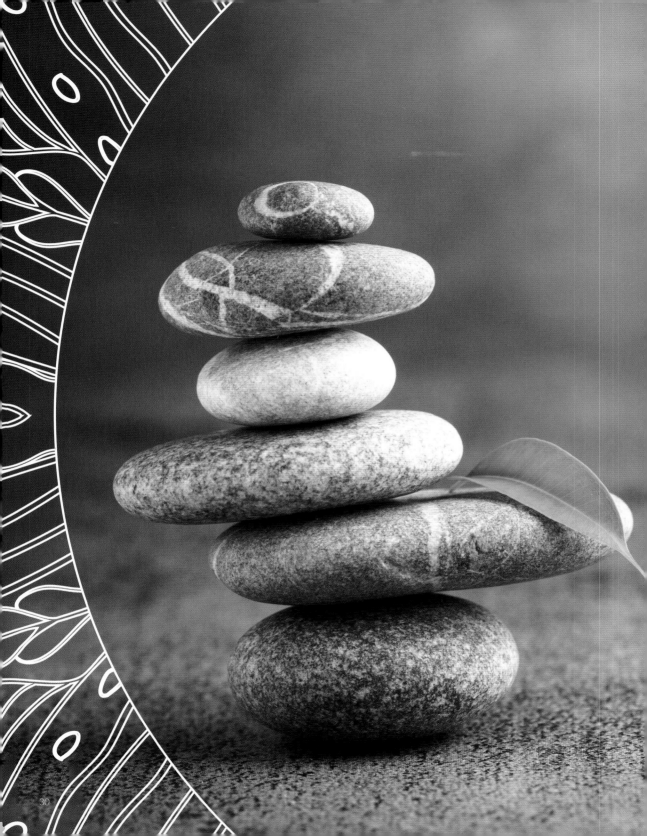

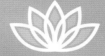

"Like any other science, yoga is applicable to people of every clime and time. Yoga is a method for restraining the natural turbulence of thoughts, which otherwise impartially prevent all men, of all lands, from glimpsing their true nature. Yoga cannot know a barrier of East and West any more than does the healing and equitable light of the sun. So long as man possesses a mind with its restless thoughts, so long will there be a universal need for yoga."

— Paramahansa Yogananda

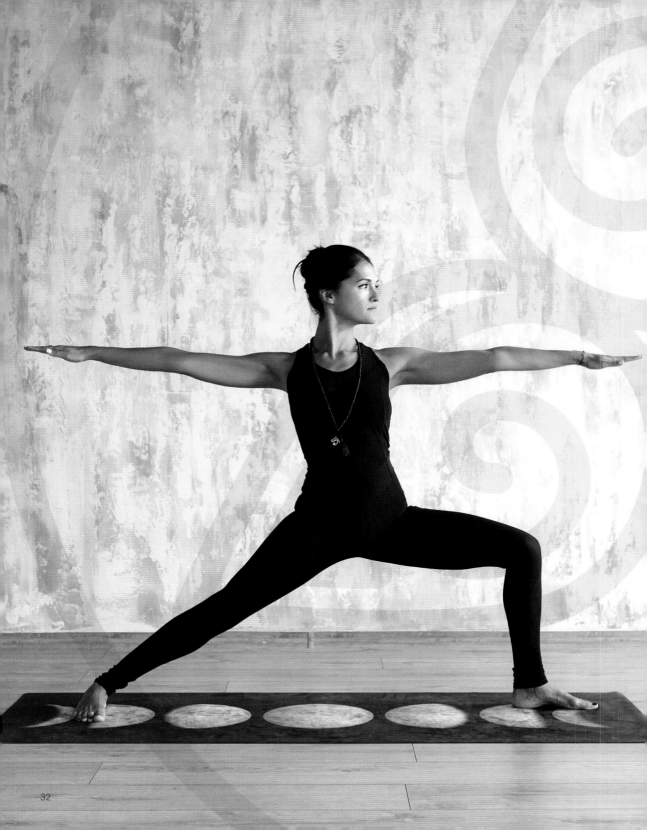

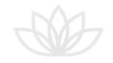

Warrior 2

Warrior 2 pose is a leg stretch, a very mild balance exercise, and an arm endurance exercise all in one. Start with your feet wide. Turn your front foot forward and parallel with the long edges of the mat and your back foot turned in slightly. Line your front heel up with the arch of your back foot. Bend your front knee and have your knee lined up directly over your front ankle. Relax your front toes and ground through the back edge of your back foot. Stretch your arms out, parallel to the floor, forming one long line through your shoulders. Keep your shoulders over your hips as you gaze over your front fingers.

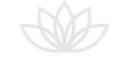

Reverse Warrior

Reverse warrior is a side stretch and a very mild balance exercise. From warrior 2 pose, keep the original shape of your legs as you flip your front palm and reach your arm up and over your head, fingers reaching back. Simultaneously slide your back hand down the side of your back leg. Your back hand will rest on the side of your thigh or possibly your shin. Feel the side of your body lengthen as you stretch, forming a crescent through your back leg and staying rooted through your feet. If you struggle to balance, bring your feet closer together and reduce the bend in your front knee, creating a more stable base.

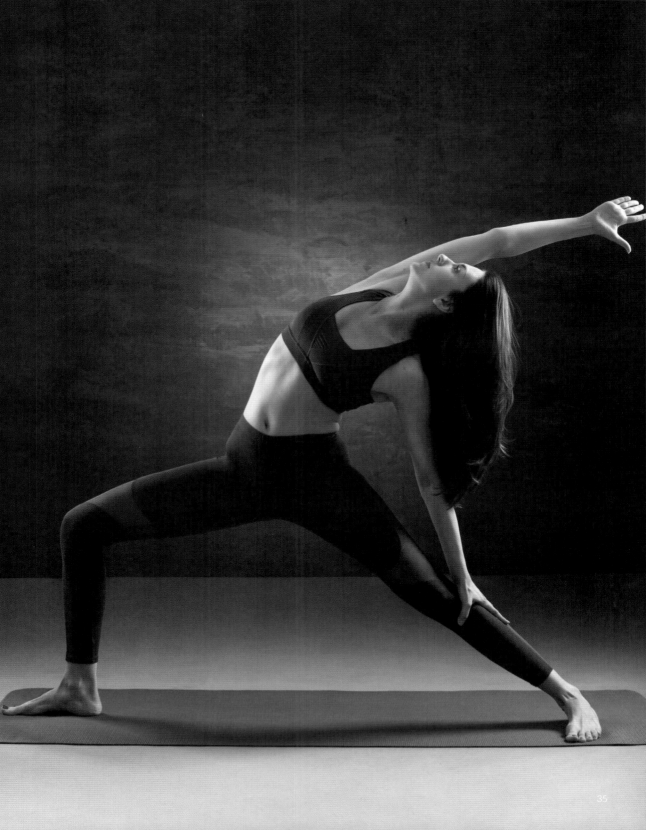

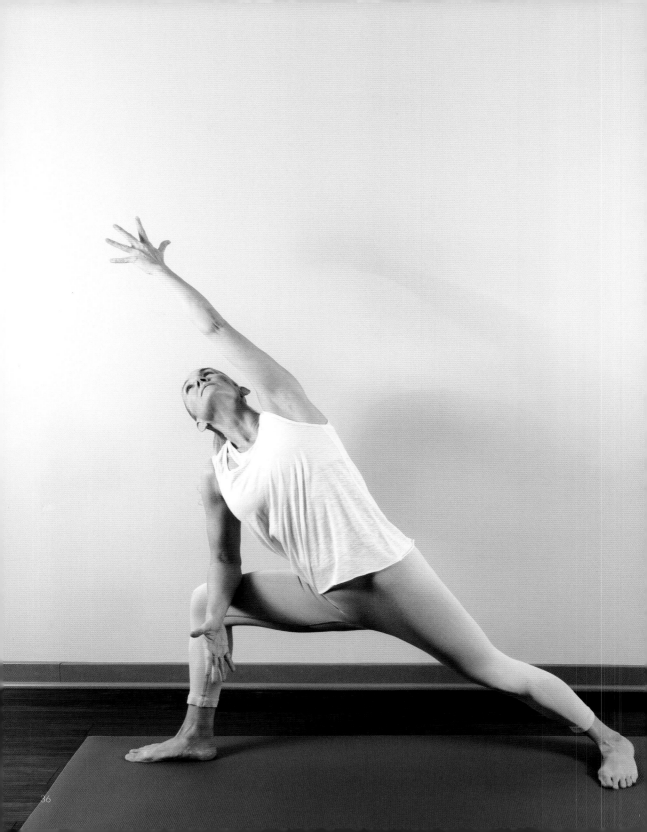

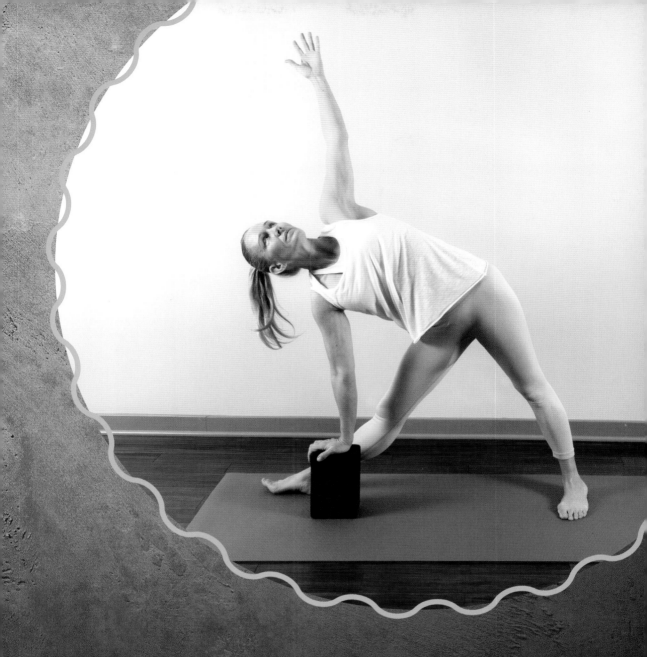

front foot. Simultaneously reach your other arm straight up toward the ceiling, stacking one shoulder over the other. Turn your gaze toward your upper hand, or allow your neck to relax if it is more comfortable. You can shorten your stance or use a yoga block beneath your front hand to help with this pose.

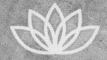

Pyramid Pose

Pyramid pose is a leg stretch with a different footing than the previous few poses. Place your feet a bit wider than your shoulders and parallel to the edges of the mat. Step one foot about 2 ½ - 3 feet behind you and angle your back toes out slightly. Place your hands on your hips and hinge forward over your

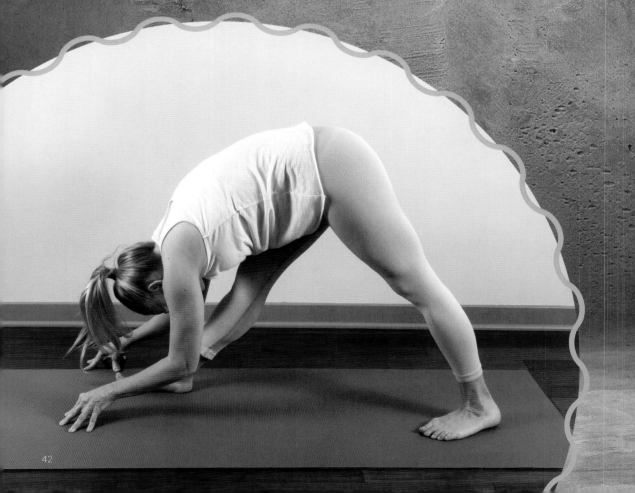

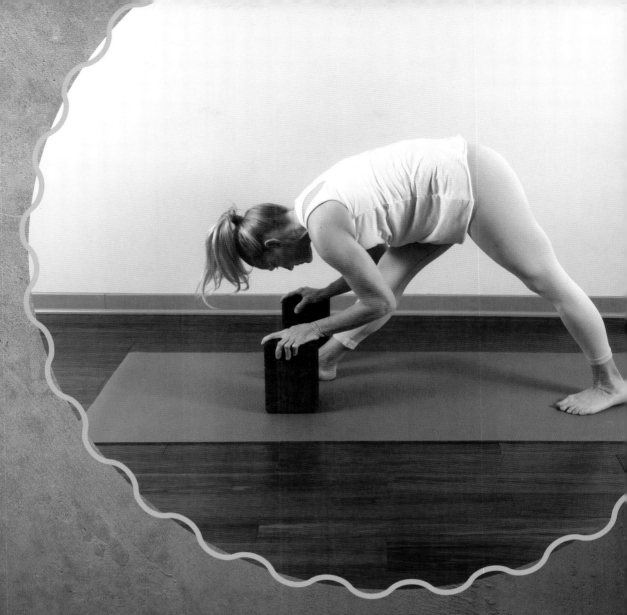

front leg, reaching your nose toward your front toes. Relax your hands to the floor or yoga blocks, on either side of your front foot. Feel the stretch on your front leg as you stay rooted through both front and back feet. Let your arms and neck relax. Breathe.

Tree pose is a body stretch and balancing exercise. Stand with your feet parallel and your hands on your hips. Find a steady gazing point on the floor or wall in front of you. Ground your weight onto one foot as you lift the opposite leg and position the foot flat against the inside of your standing leg. You can adjust this foot as low or high as is comfortable, but avoid pressing it into your knee.

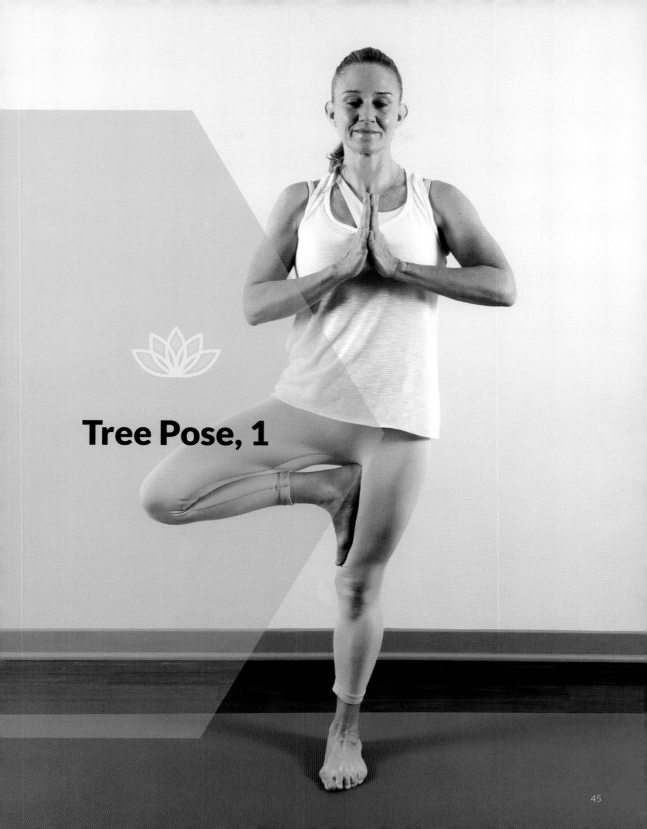

Tree Pose, 1

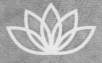

Tree Pose, 2

Once you feel secure, make sure your shoulders are positioned over your hips. Reach your arms up wide and then high overhead with your palms facing each other. When you feel steady and are comfortable, you can turn your gaze upward.

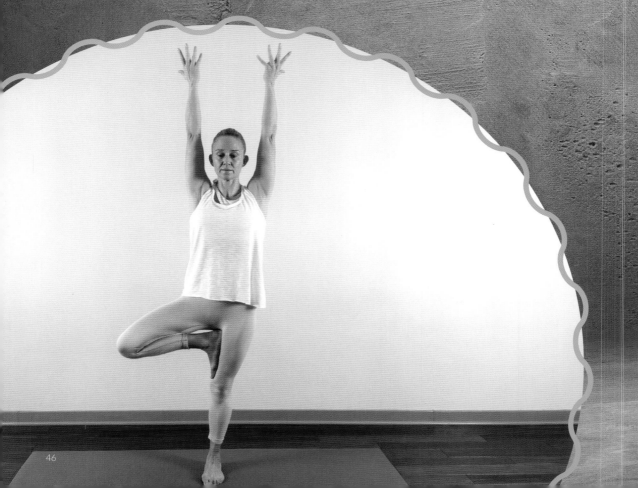

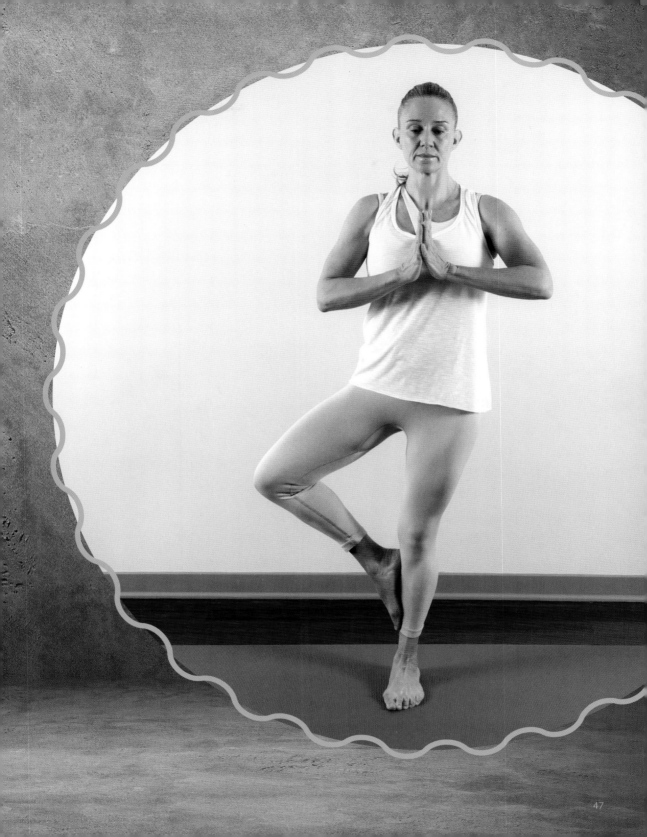

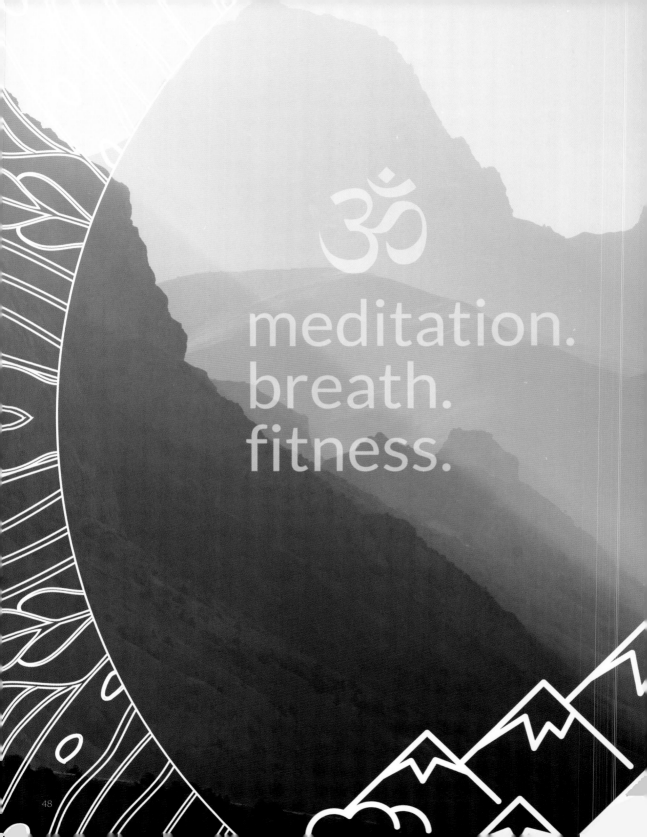

meditation.
breath.
fitness.

48

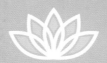

"View in yourself the soul of all beings and those beings themselves; think your own self or soul as the microcosm of the great universe, and be tolerant and broad sighted in your practice of Yoga."

— Valmiki

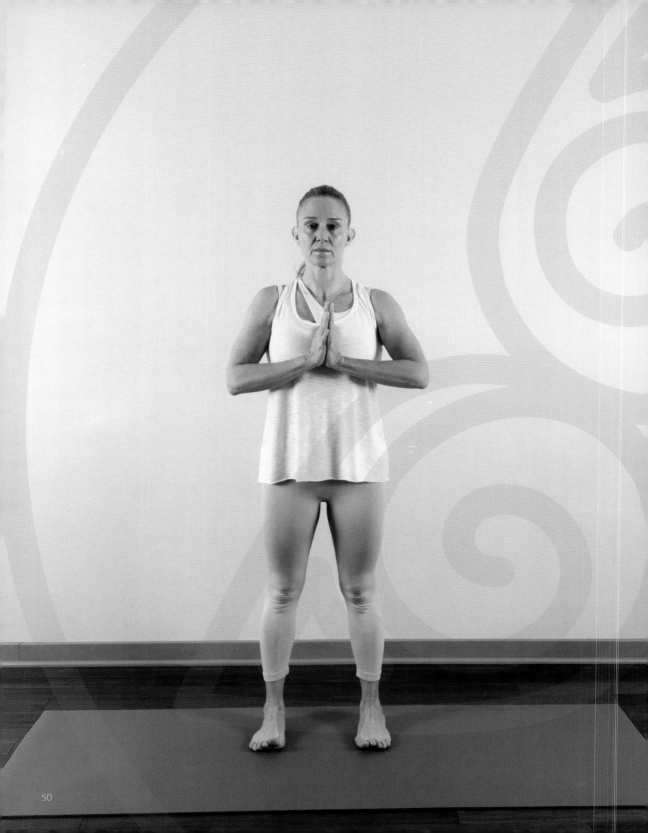

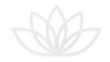

Half Sun Salutation

Half sun salutation is an active flow that begins with a symbolic hand gesture called a **mudra** (ᴍoo-druh). In mountain pose, stand with your feet hip width apart. Press your hands together and position them over the center of your chest, resting your thumbs on your sternum. Press your knuckles toward each other as you hold your fingers together or spread them apart. This hand pose is referred to as **anjali mudra**. Often, the ancient Sanskrit word **namaste** is said when this hand gesture is used at the end of a yoga class.

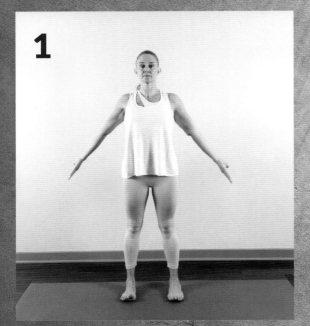

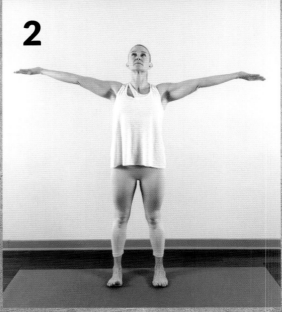

1–4. From the anjali mudra, let your hands lower and separate in front of you. Turn your palms out, let your shoulders drop, and raise your arms in a wide, intentional arc as you take a big breath in through your nose.

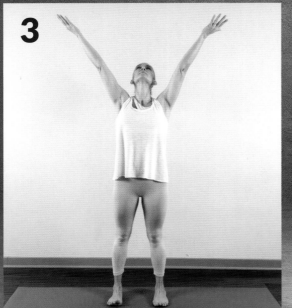

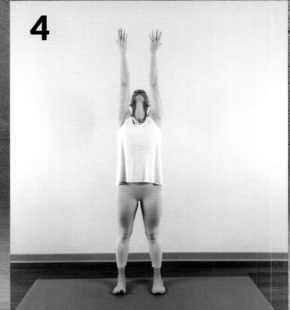

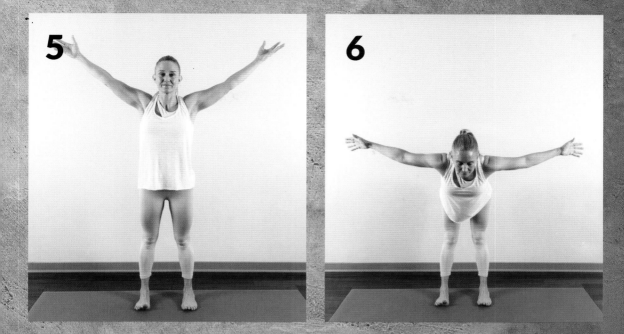

5–8. After you complete your inhale with an upward salute, begin your exhale as you start to forward fold. Turn your palms outward and hinge at the hips as you arc your arms down toward a standing forward fold.

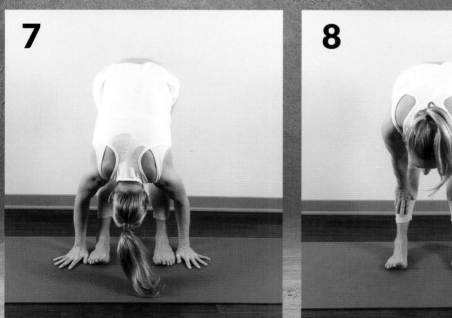
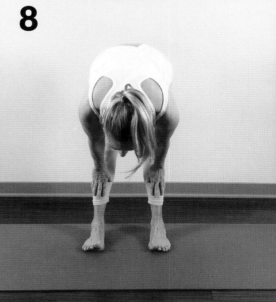

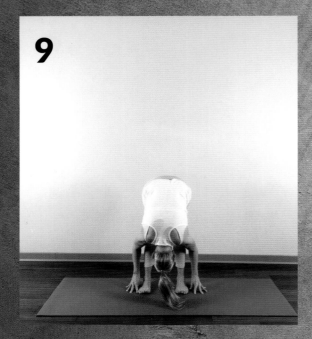

9

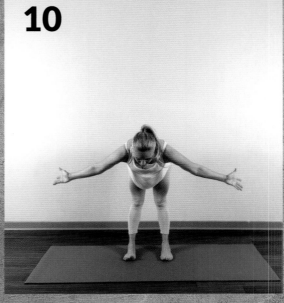

10

9–12. Exhale as you once again bend fully forward. On an inhale, lift your upper body and begin to raise your hands in a wide swing. Let your palms turn toward each other as your arms rise. Bring your gaze upward.

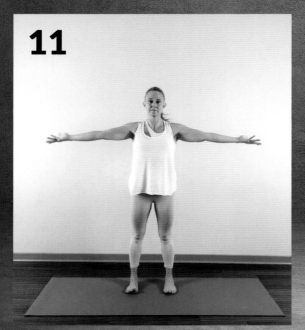

11

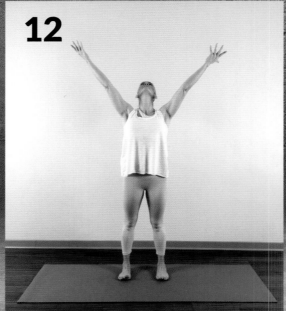

12

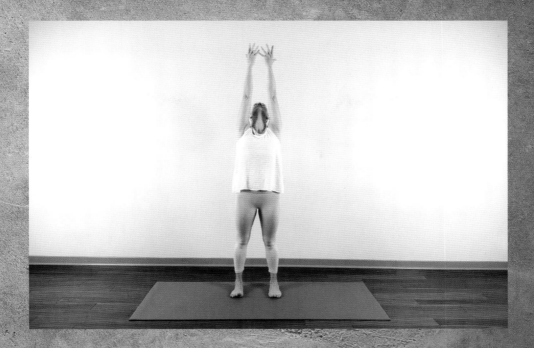

Finish. As you complete your inhale, reach completely upward toward the ceiling as you gaze toward your fingers. Finally, on an exhale, finish the flow by letting your arms drop and return to the center of your chest.

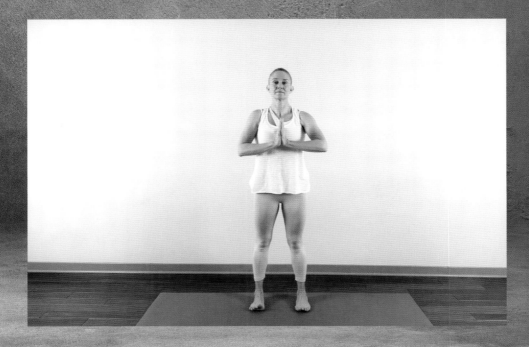

Seated Poses

EASY SEATED POSE • TWIST VARIATION •
SIDE STRETCH • BUTTERFLY • STAFF POSE •
SEATED FORWARD FOLD • HEAD TO KNEE •
HALF LORD OF THE FISHES • NECK ROLL

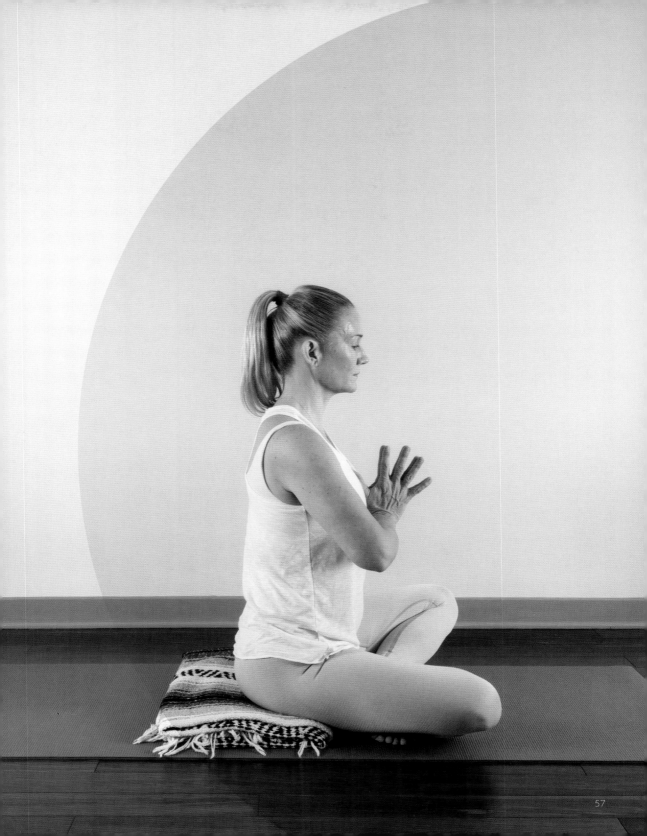

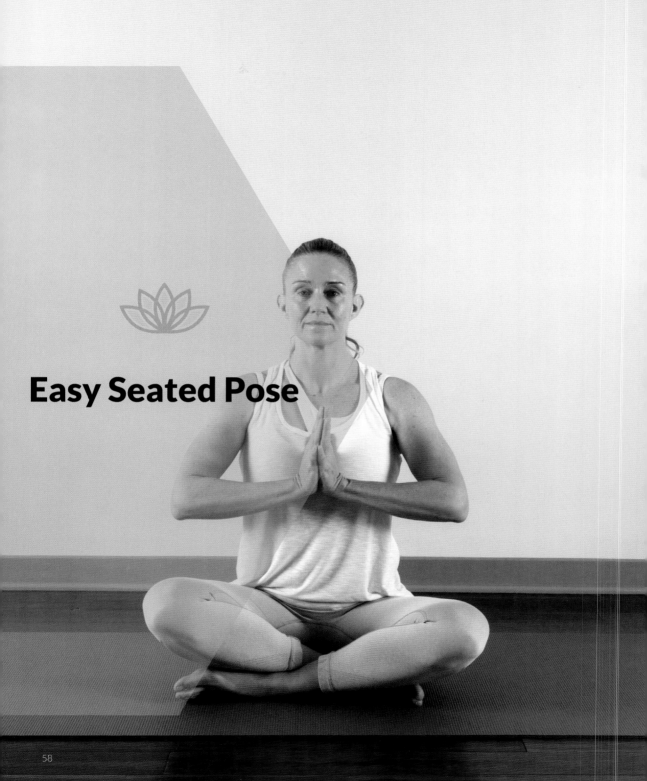

Easy Seated Pose

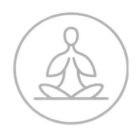

Easy seated pose is a simple grounding exercise. Sit with your legs crossed to whatever extent is comfortable. You can use folded blankets or a yoga block to lift your hips, or sit on a firm cushion like a bolster. Lengthen your spine as you bring your shoulders up toward your ears and then roll them down your back, bringing your shoulder blades closer together. Feel your chest lift. Reach the the top of your head toward the ceiling as your spine lengthens. Bring your hands together at the center of your chest as you take long, slow inhales and exhales. Turn your thoughts toward gratitude.

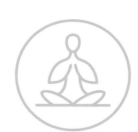

You can create a spinal twist from easy seated pose. Place one hand on the opposite knee as pictured, and your other hand to the floor or a yoga block behind your back as you gently twist. Keep your hips grounded as you twist only as much as is comfortable. Inhale as you lengthen your spine upward and exhale as you twist more. Avoid pushing or straining as you turn your gaze over your back shoulder. Allow your body to tell you when to stop, then return to your seated position. Repeat for the other side.

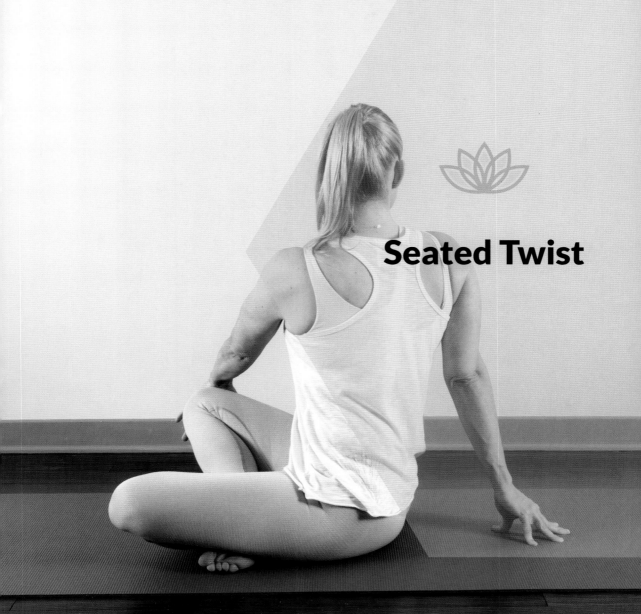

Seated Twist

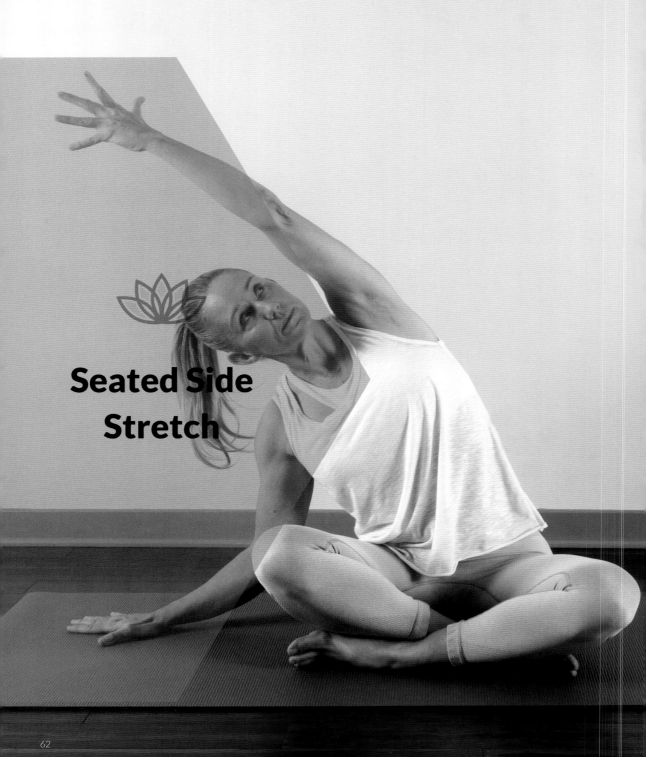

Seated Side
Stretch

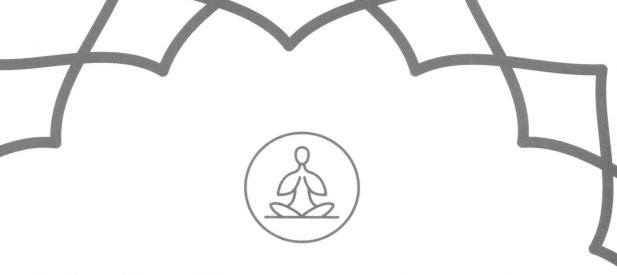

Creating a side stretch from easy seated pose is an effective way to lengthen and stretch your upper body. Similarly to grounding through your feet in a standing pose, allow your "sitting bones" to ground you into your seat. Reach one hand out to the side beyond your hip, then stretch your opposite arm up and over your head, palm facing down. Feel your side lengthen as you breathe in and out. You can relax your neck or turn to look toward the ceiling, as your chest turns upward. Root down into your hips and lift back to the start, then repeat for the other side.

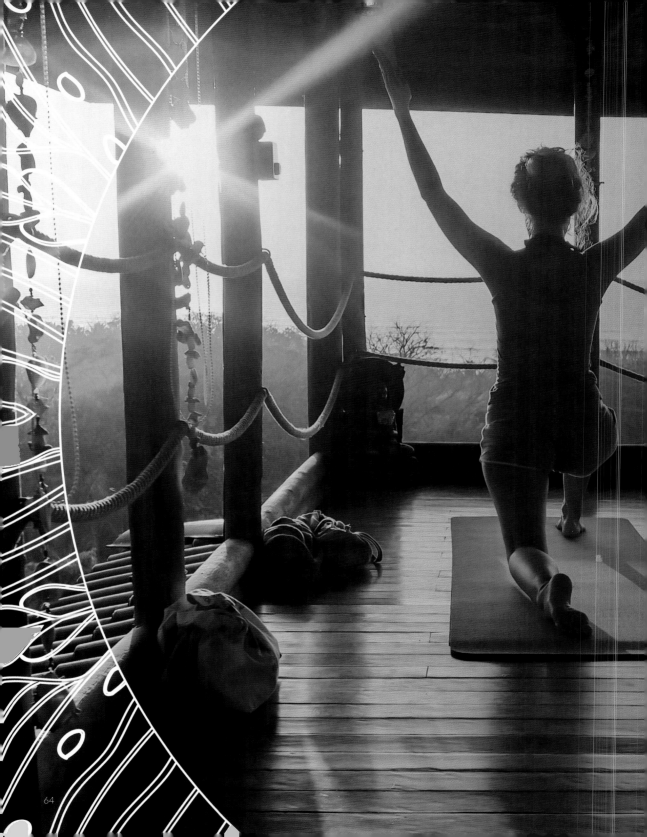

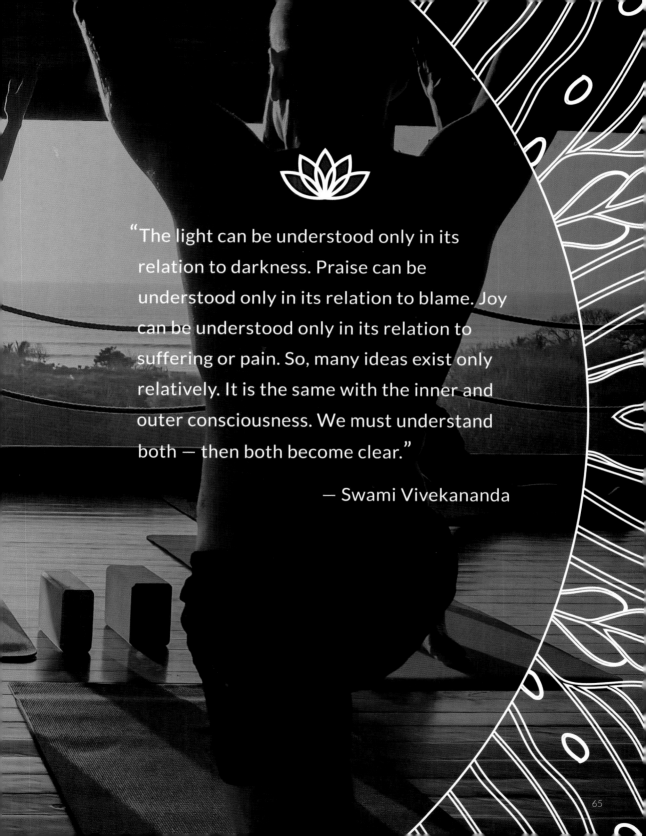

"The light can be understood only in its relation to darkness. Praise can be understood only in its relation to blame. Joy can be understood only in its relation to suffering or pain. So, many ideas exist only relatively. It is the same with the inner and outer consciousness. We must understand both — then both become clear."

— Swami Vivekananda

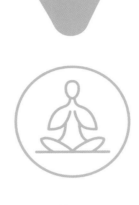

Butterfly pose is an excellent stretch for your hips and your low back. Place the soles of your feet together, and hold your calves, ankles or feet with your hands. Bring your heels as far inward as is comfortable, and let your bent knees drop softly toward the floor. You can use blankets, blocks, or a bolster to help support you. Feel the stretch as you let your shoulders drop and you lean forward slightly.

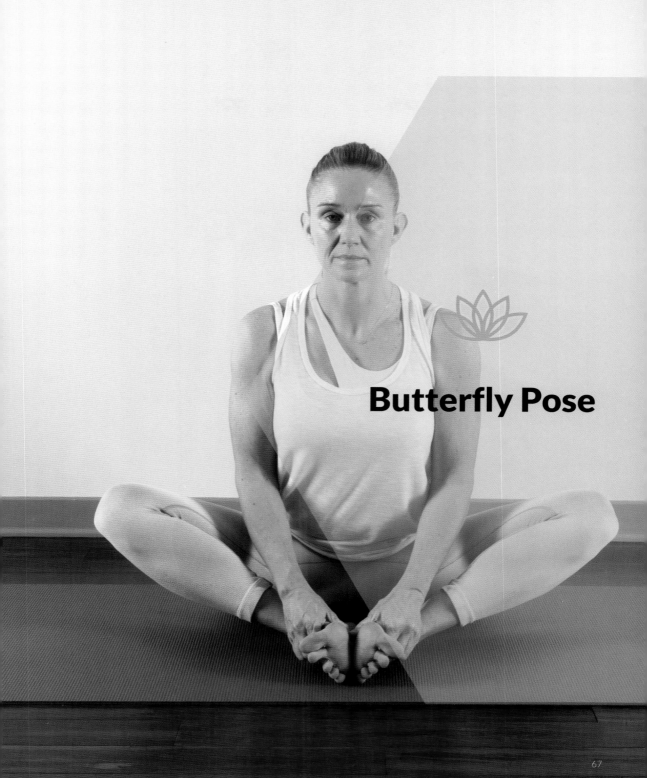

Butterfly Pose

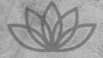

Butterfly Pose

As a variation, you can sit upright with your hands resting on the floor or yoga blocks behind your back. Feel the tension in your hips relax as you soften your jaw and breathe into the stretch.

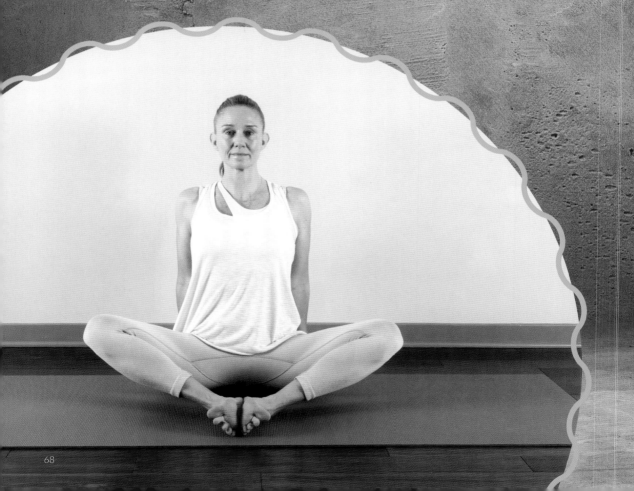

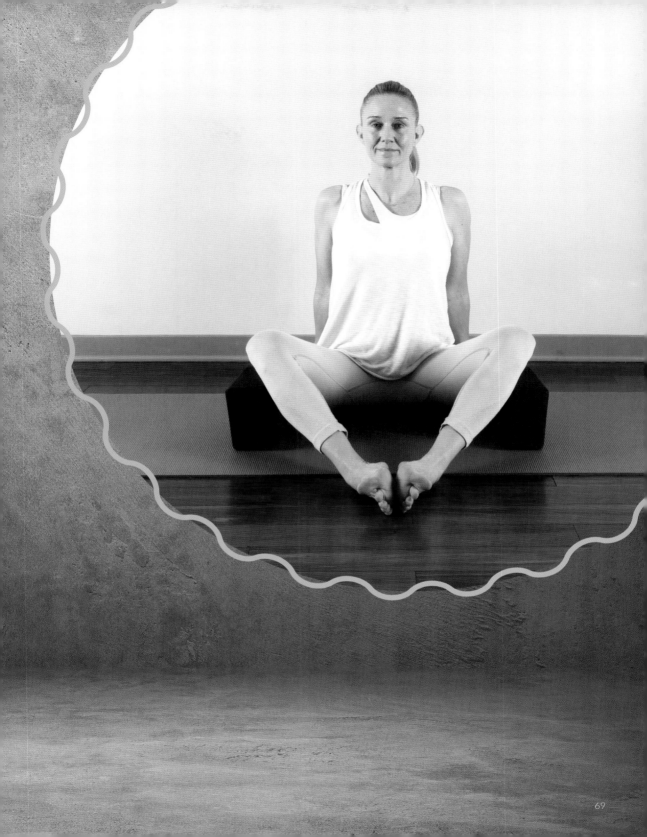

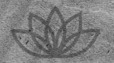

Staff Pose

Staff pose is the seated version of mountain pose, in terms of wonderful posture and alignment for your spine. Sit with your legs in front of you and flex your feet with toes pointing up. Rest your hands on your thighs or to the floor beside your hips

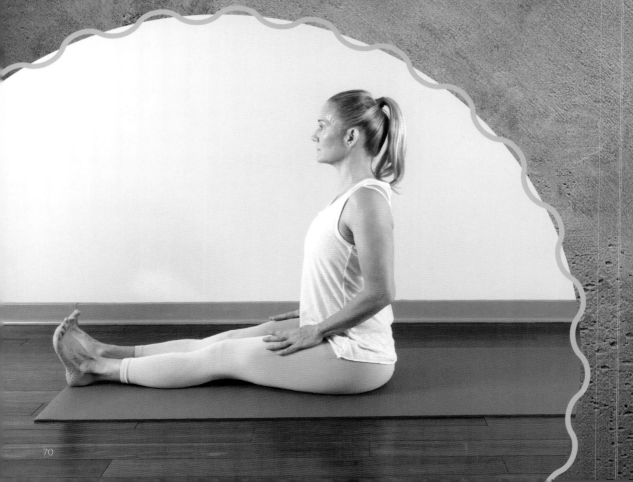

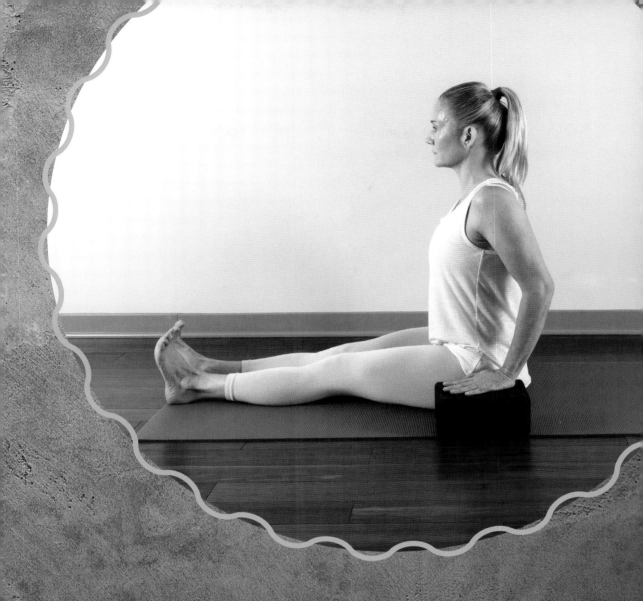

and feel your sitting bones grounding you. Breathe in and roll your shoulders up, back and down, feeling your spine lengthen and relax as you support it with your breath. Feel your chest lift as you breathe and lengthen. You can use yoga blocks to support your hands or a folded blanket beneath your hips or your knees to make sure you are comfortable and your shoulders are positioned on top of your hips.

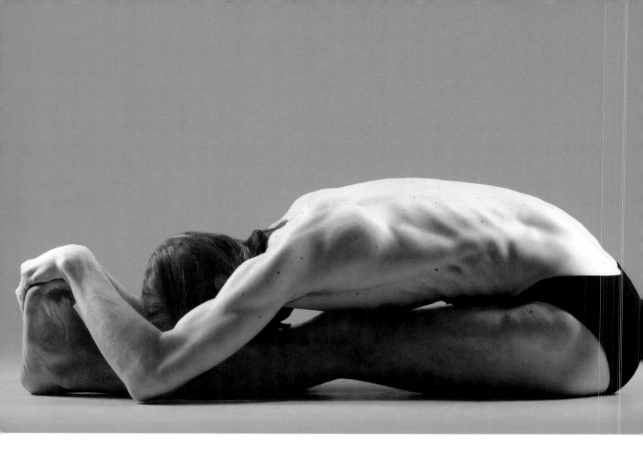

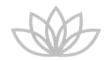

Seated Forward Fold

Seated forward fold pose is the seated version of standing forward fold, providing a wonderful stretch for the back of your legs and your low back.

Begin in staff pose with your legs parallel as you lift your arms straight up above your head. Feel your spine lengthen from your tailbone all the way up through

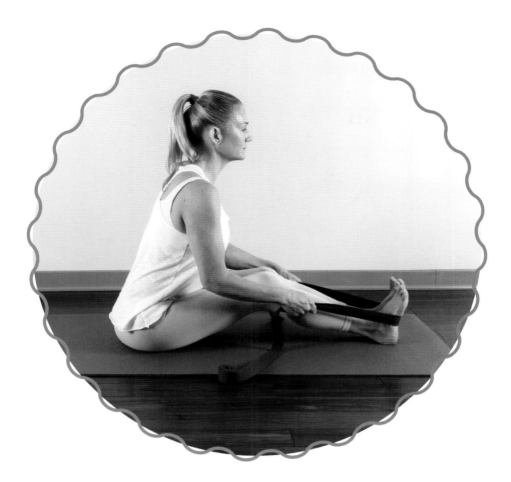

the top of your head. Fold forward as you hinge from your hips and reach toward your toes. You can bend your knees or use a strap to get an effective stretch if it is difficult to touch your toes. If desired, sit on a few blankets to elevate your hips. Focus your gaze above your toes as you take smooth and steady inhales and exhales.

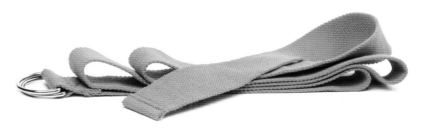

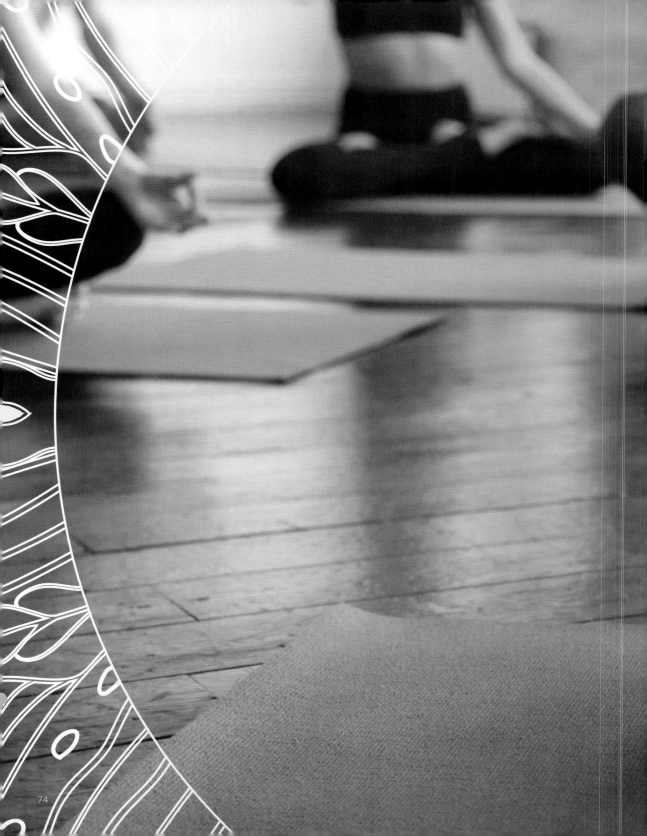

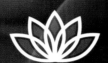

"Student! Your life is your own. You have only yourself to thank for what you are, have been and will be. Take your present into your own hand. Consciously shape out of it your future."

— A.P. Mukerji

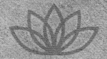

Head to Knee Pose

Head to knee pose is the seated version of tree pose, offering a nice stretch for your hips, hamstrings and spine. Begin in staff pose with both legs forward, then bring one leg in to form a triangle. Your upper body will twist slightly as you fold over

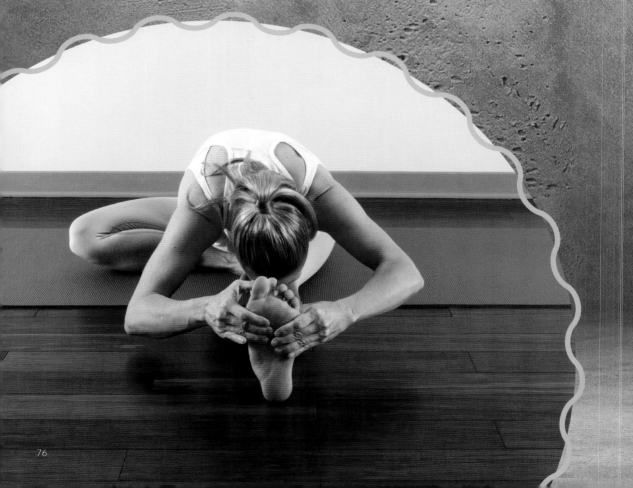

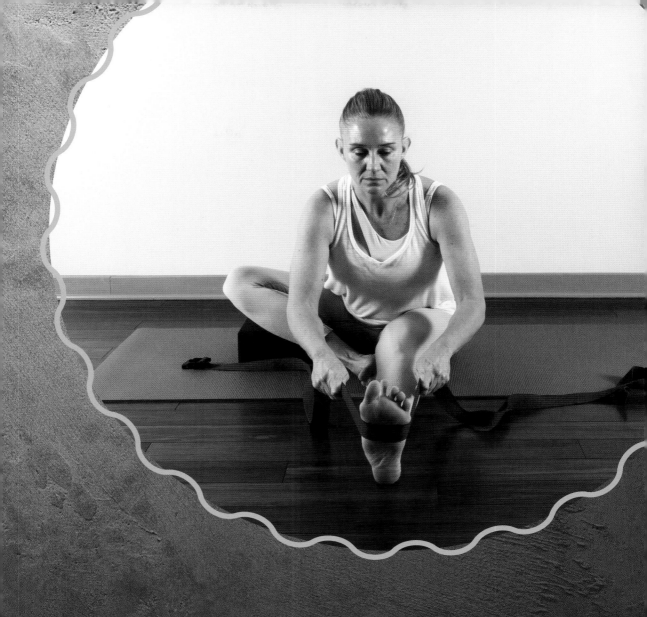

your extended leg and reach for your foot, ankle or shin. Keep a slight bend in your extended leg or use a strap to help you. Turn your gaze over your toes or close your eyes as you take several deep breaths. Feel your spine lengthen as you stretch. Use your hands to lift you up to a seated position and switch sides.

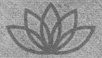

Half Lord of the Fishes

Half lord of the fishes pose is a gentle seated twist for your spine and core. Begin in staff pose with both legs forward, then bend the knee on one leg and place your foot firmly outside or inside your extended leg. Bring your arm from your

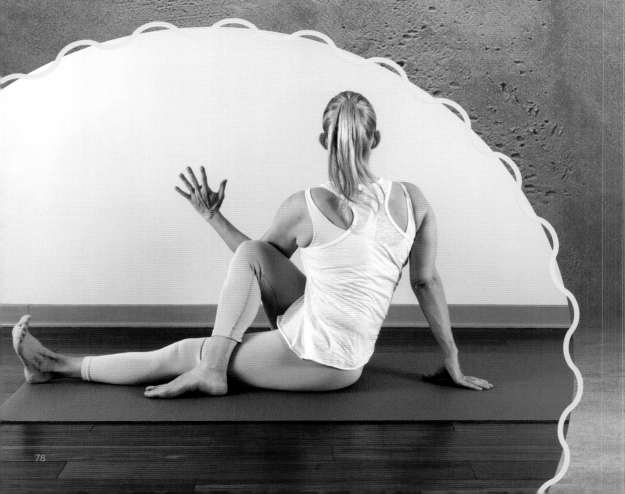

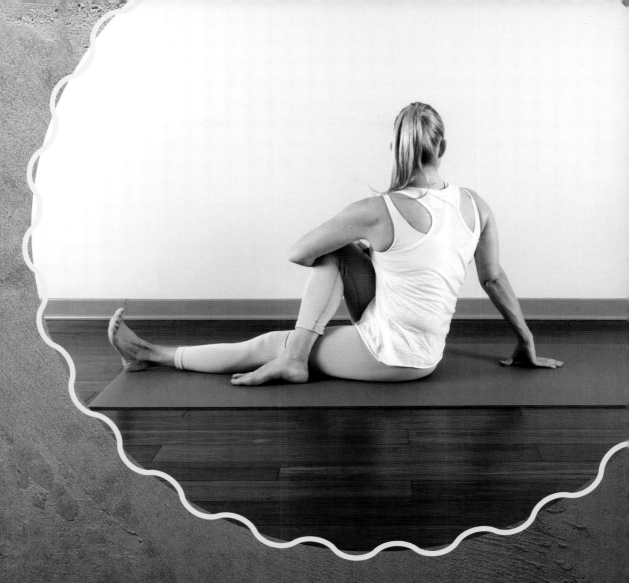

bent leg side behind you as you lift your other arm toward the ceiling and stretch your side long. Twist at the waist and rotate your body until you can settle your opposite elbow or hand on your bent leg as pictured. Inhale as you lengthen your spine upward and exhale as you twist further. Release the stretch and return to neutral, then uncross your legs and pause for a breath. Repeat for the opposite side.

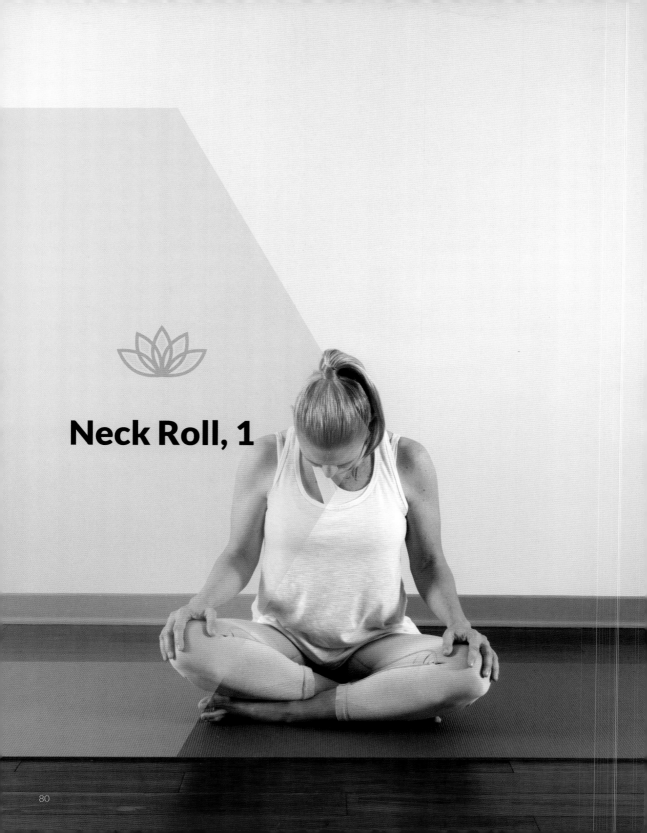

Neck Roll, 1

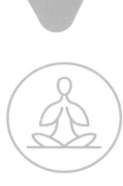

The neck roll is a classic stretching exercise that also helps to lengthen your spine and center you in your practice. Sit with legs crossed in easy seated pose, and rest your hands on your knees. If this is uncomfortable, you can open your legs and lift your hips on folded blankets, a cushion or a yoga block. Roll your shoulders up, back and down as you lengthen your spine and ground through your sitting bones. Drop your chin to your chest and breathe into the stretch on the back of your neck.

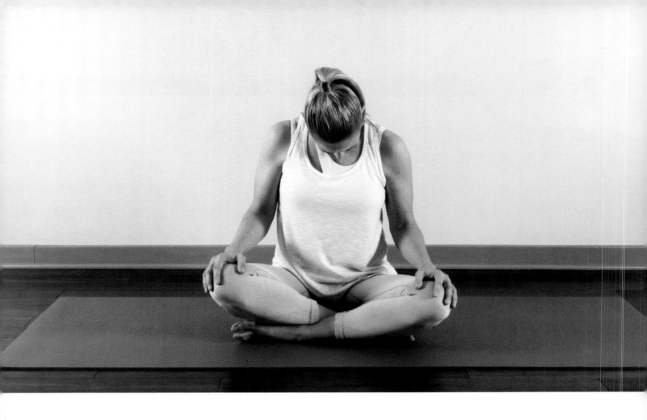

Neck Roll, 2

Keep your sitting bones settled on the floor. Rotate your neck, making a smooth arc of steady and intentional motion. Keep the rest of your body as still and neutral as you can. Finally, return your head to the beginning position, resting against your chest. Feel how much looser and less resistant your neck muscles are. If it is uncomfortable to make full rotations with your neck, keep your head in front of your body and sway your head left to right. Bring your head back up to a neutral position and rest for a moment while you breathe.

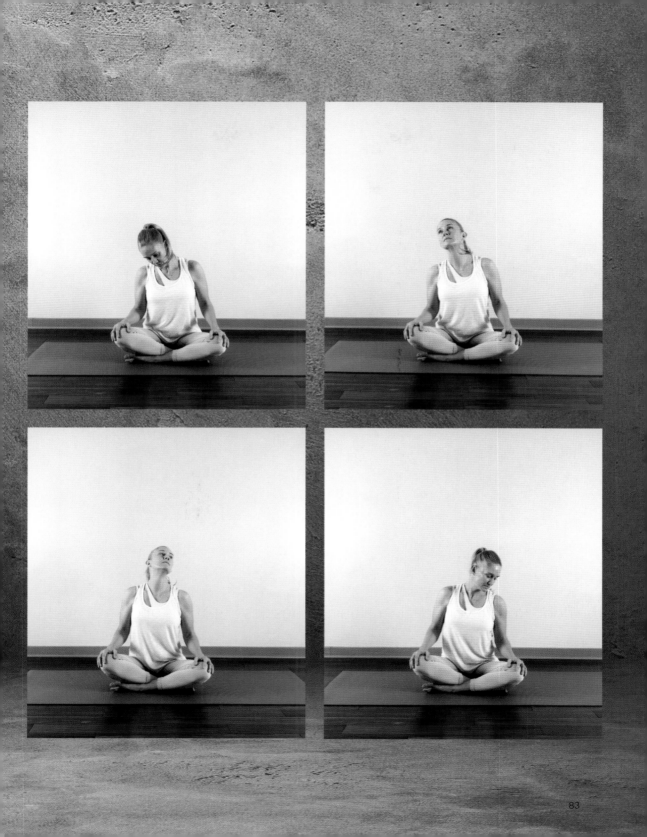

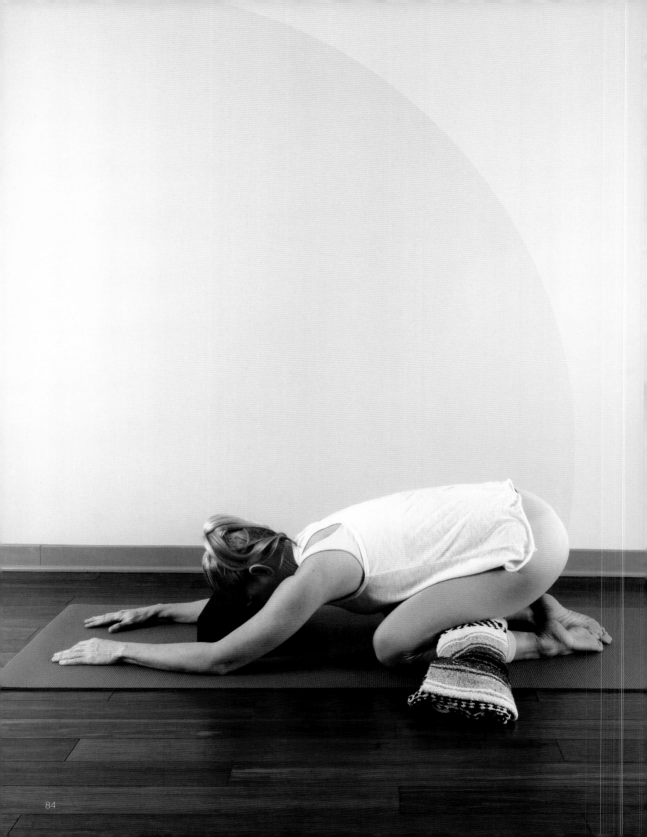

Prone Poses

CHILD'S POSE • TABLE • SPINAL BALANCE •
PUPPY • DOWNWARD FACING DOG • SPHYNX •
LOCUST • COBRA • GATE POSE • LOW LUNGE
• HALF SPLITS

Child's Pose

Child's pose is considered to be a resting pose between other, more active postures. If you feel sensitivity in your knees, cushion your knees with a blanket or roll a blanket up and place it behind your knees. Bring your shins parallel on the mat or knees wide as you use your hands to press your hips toward your heels. If your forehead does not reach the floor, rest your head on a yoga block to avoid straining your neck, pictured on page 89.

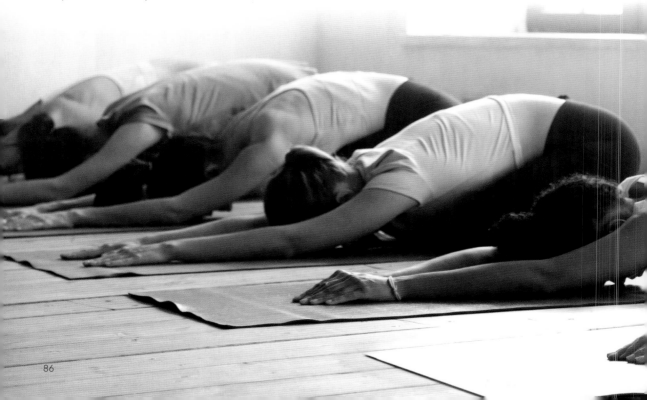

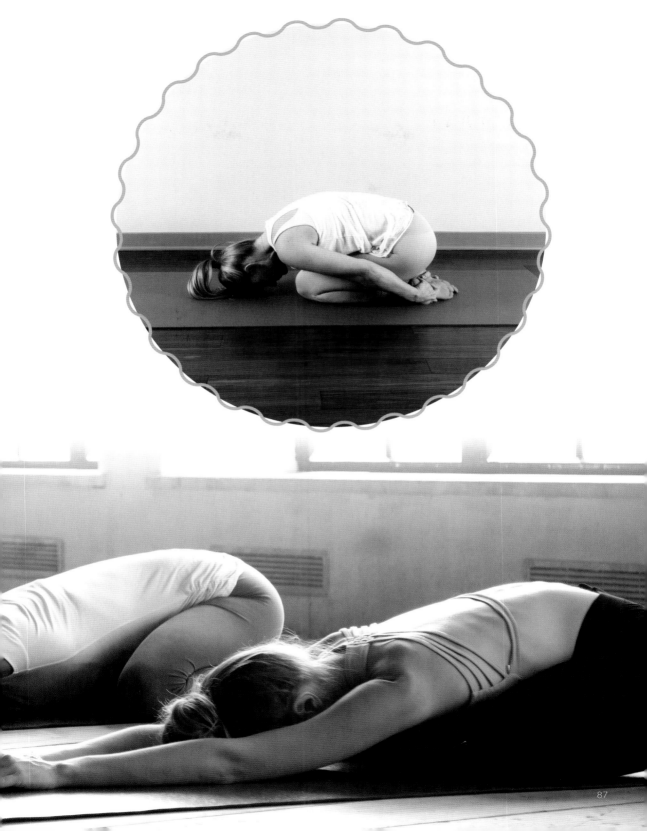

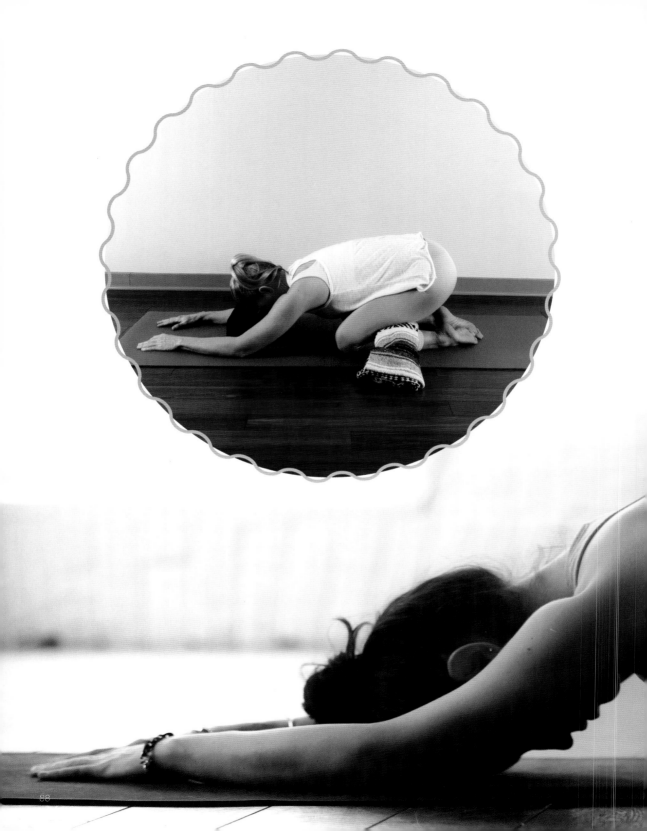

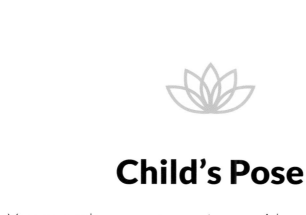

Child's Pose

You can relax your arms at your sides or reach your hands forward, pictured on the facing page, into a more active version of the pose.

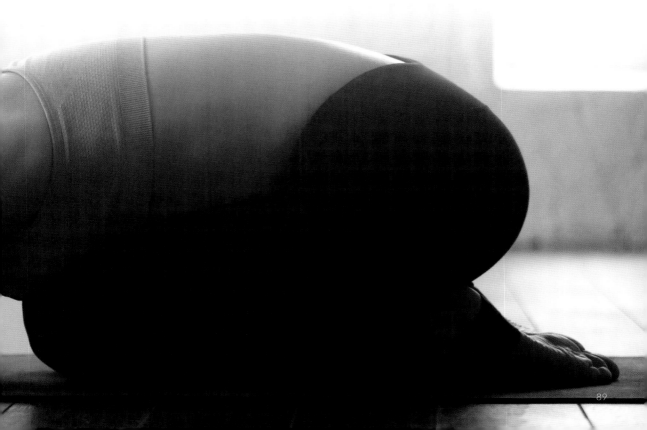

Table Pose

Table pose is a neutral posture from which you can move into various other poses. Start with your hands and feet shoulder width apart, forming 90° angles to your upper body. Align your shoulders on top of your hands and your hips on top of your

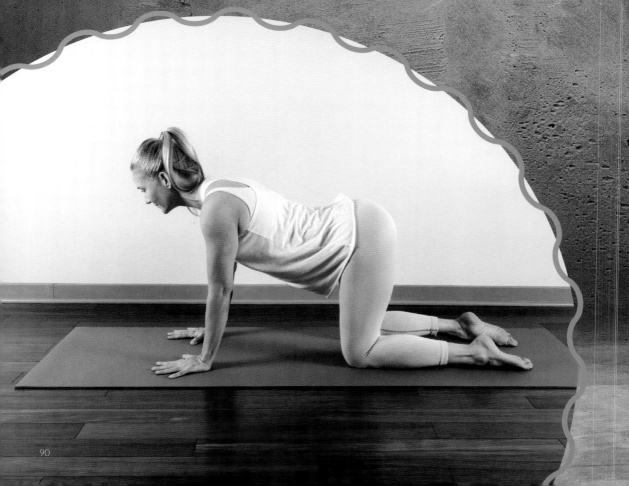

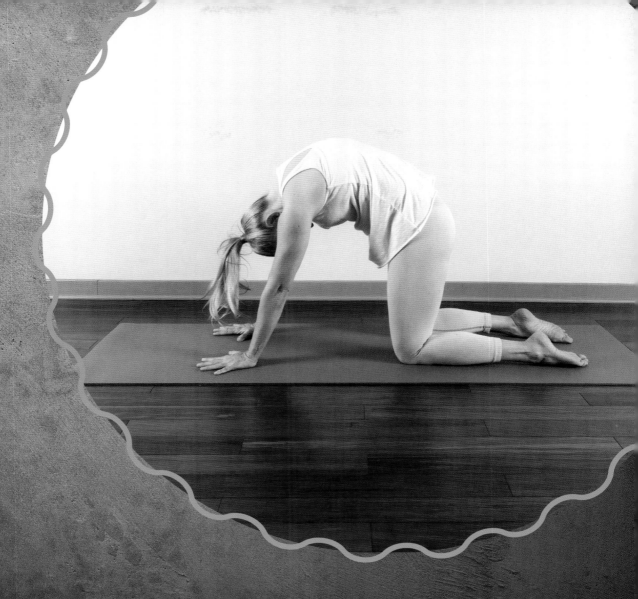

knees, with parallel shins. If you
have knee sensitivity, place a
blanket under your knees. Keep
your spine neutral, rooting through
your hands and spreading your
fingers wide. Press your shins and
the tops of your feet into the floor.

From there, you can roll your spine
into a U shape, inhaling as you do.
This is cow pose. Exhale as you roll
your spine back up into an arch.
This is cat pose. Flow through cat
and cow pose as you follow your
breath.

Spinal Balance

Spinal balance is a challenging pose that combines strength, stretching and core work. Begin in table pose with a neutral spine. Raise one arm and the opposite leg until both are parallel to the floor with your toes flexed down and your palm faced inward. Keep your head in line with your spine. Hold the

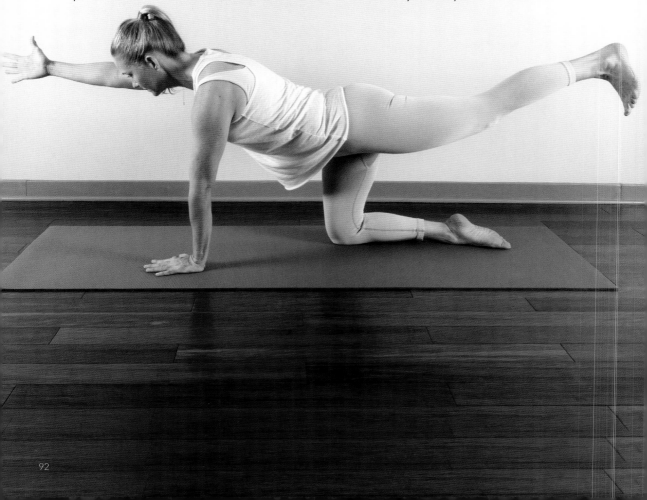

pose for a few breaths as your stretch from your fingertips through your opposite heel. Relax and lower your arm and leg back into table pose, then repeat with the opposite arm and leg. If you find this pose to be too challenging, you can lower your leg and rest your toes on the mat.

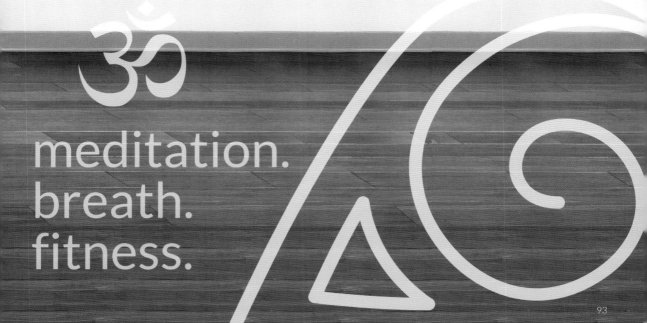

meditation.
breath.
fitness.

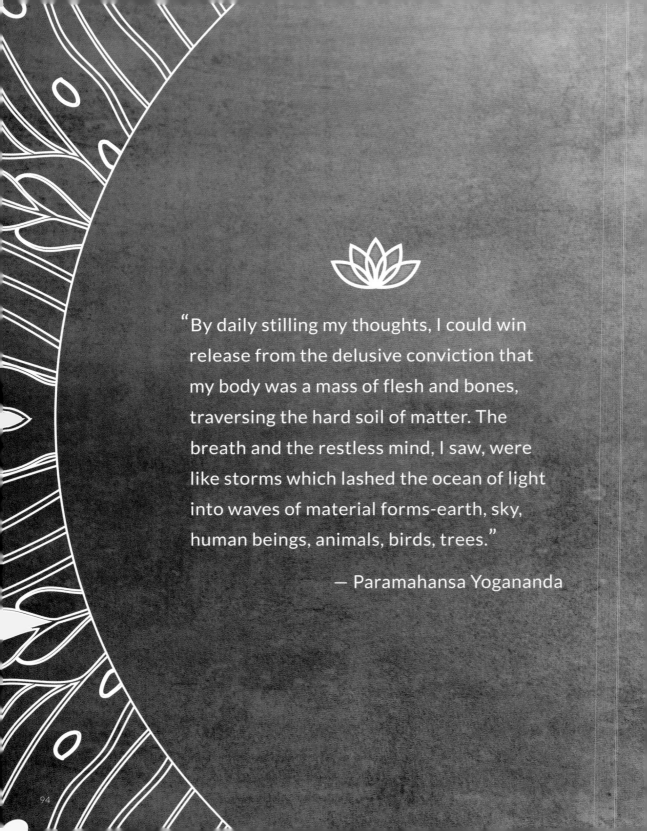

"By daily stilling my thoughts, I could win release from the delusive conviction that my body was a mass of flesh and bones, traversing the hard soil of matter. The breath and the restless mind, I saw, were like storms which lashed the ocean of light into waves of material forms-earth, sky, human beings, animals, birds, trees."

— Paramahansa Yogananda

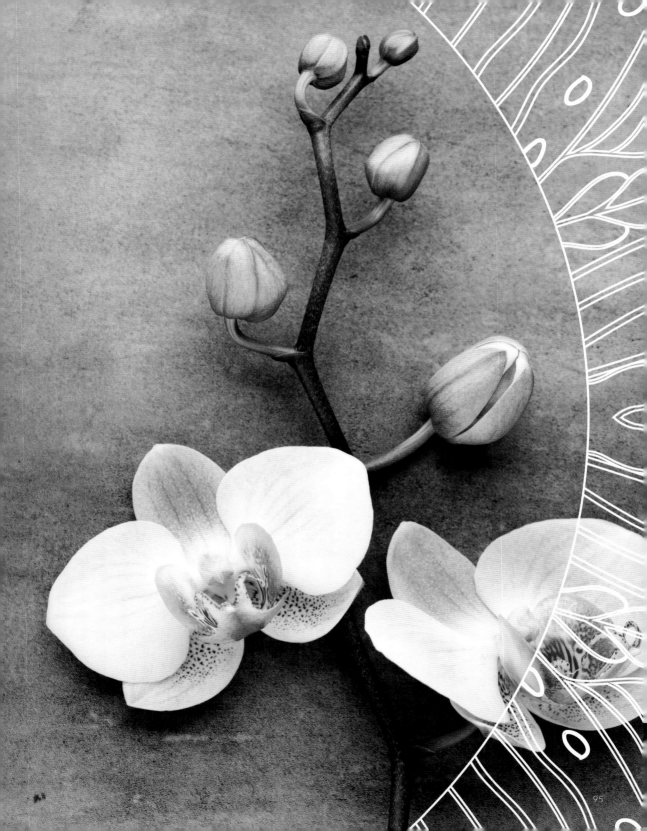

Puppy Pose

Puppy pose is a spinal backbend that starts from table pose. Keep your hips stationary over your knees as you walk your hands forward and rest your forehead on the floor or a yoga block. Keep your hips stable and above your knees as your chest drops

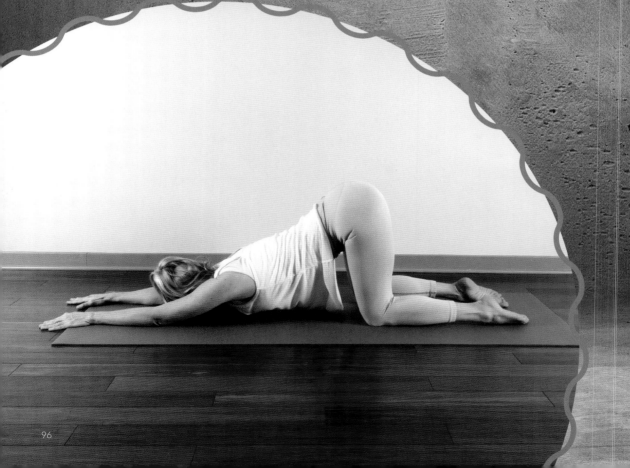

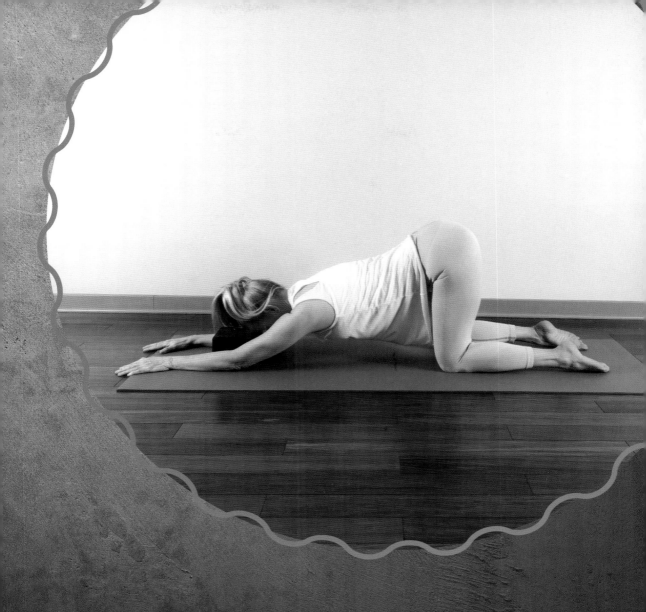

toward the floor. Press your shins and the tops of your feet flat against the floor if you can, and let your arms relax as your shoulders stretch and lengthen along with your spine. You can make this pose more active by reaching your hands further forward. Feel your back stretch and loosen, continuing to breathe.

Downward Facing Dog

Downward facing dog is a challenging pose that energizes and strengthens the entire body. Start in table pose with your fingers wide and hands firmly grounded into the mat. Move your knees back a couple of inches and come to the balls of

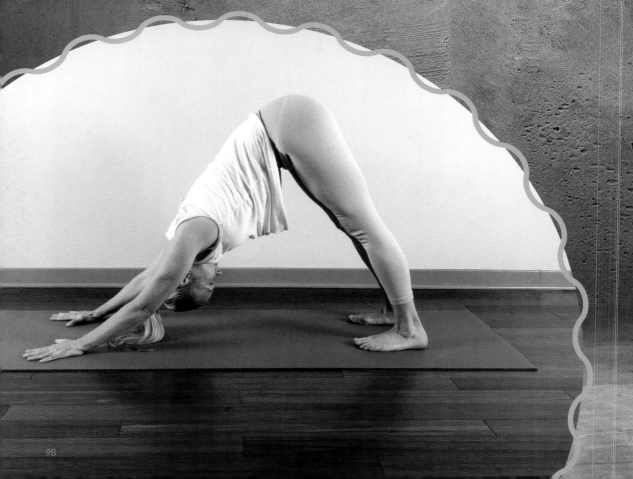

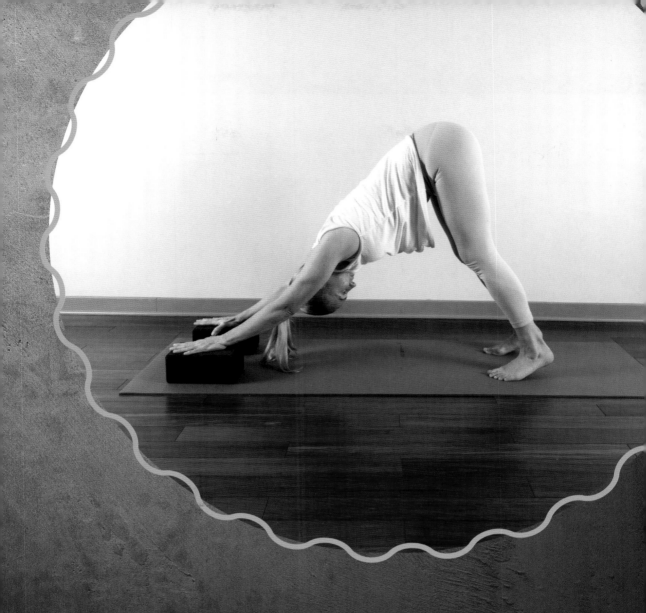

your feet as you lift your hips. Keep your legs straight but with a gentle bend in your knees. You may use blocks under your hands to assist you, as shown above. Look through your legs to the wall behind you and let your neck relax. Feel the entire back of your body lengthen, from hands to heels. Take several deep inhales and exhales as you hold the pose.

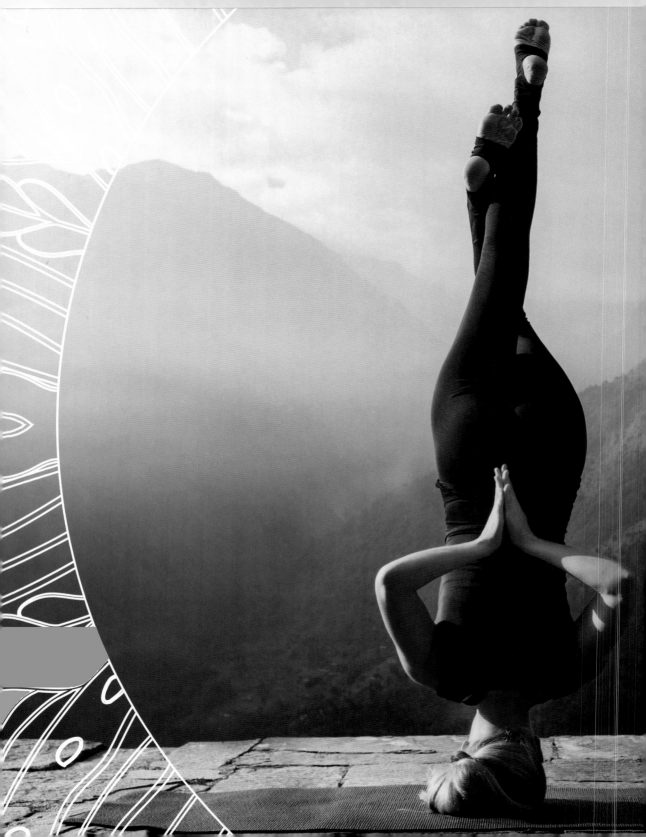

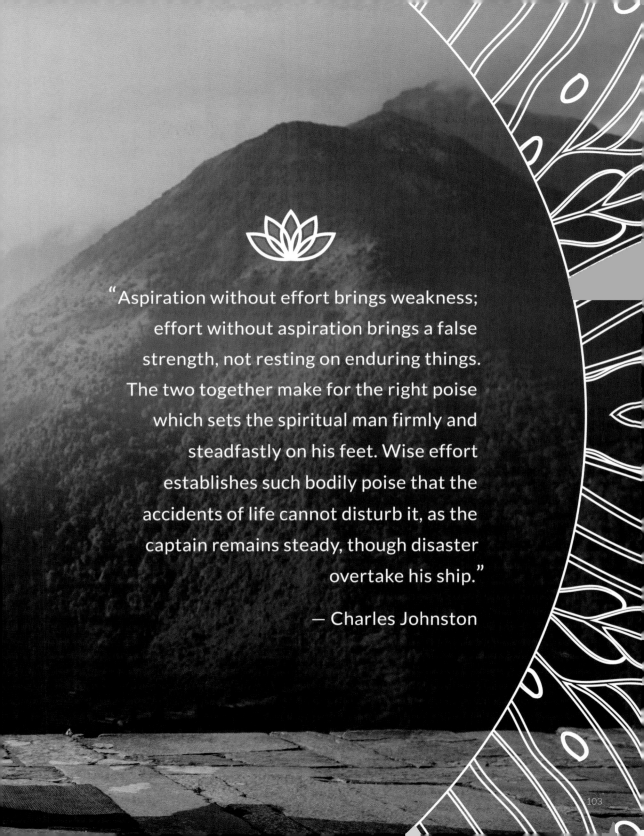

"Aspiration without effort brings weakness; effort without aspiration brings a false strength, not resting on enduring things. The two together make for the right poise which sets the spiritual man firmly and steadfastly on his feet. Wise effort establishes such bodily poise that the accidents of life cannot disturb it, as the captain remains steady, though disaster overtake his ship."

— Charles Johnston

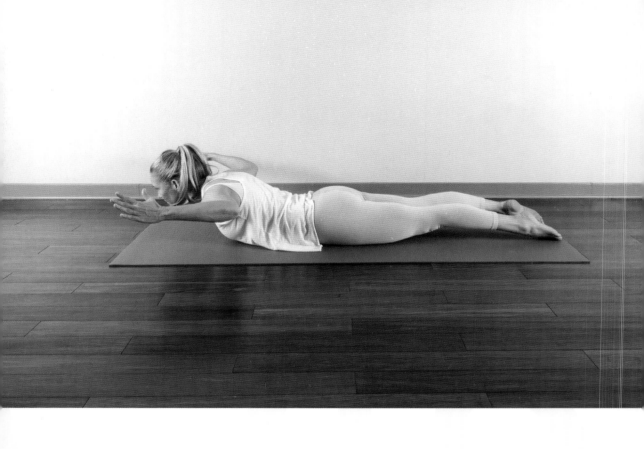

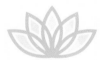

Locust Pose

Locust pose is a deeper belly backbend than sphinx pose and strengthens your entire back and legs. Lie flat on your belly and rest your forehead on the mat as you bring your arms into a "goalpost" shape. Lift your arms first as you bring your forearms parallel to the floor and your elbows in line with your shoulders, hugging your shoulder blades closer together. Engage your back muscles to lift your upper body as your gaze focuses slightly in front of your mat. Avoid straining your neck as you lift up. You can keep your legs on the mat or lift them up as well, bringing your inner thighs together and perhaps spreading your toes.

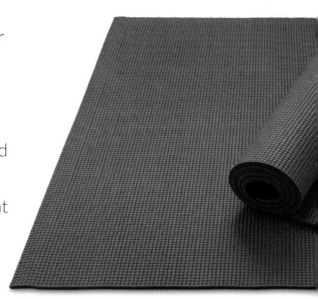

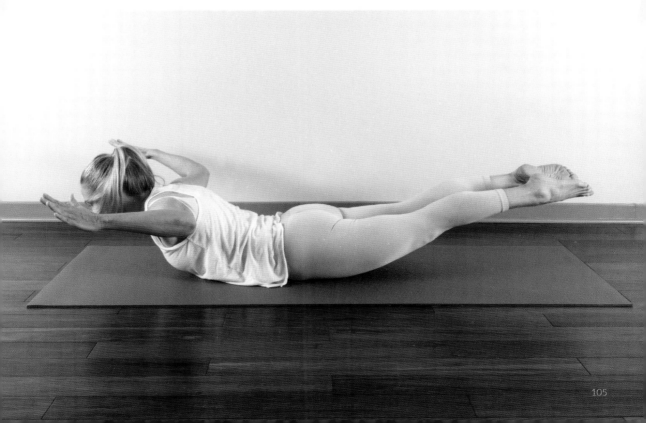

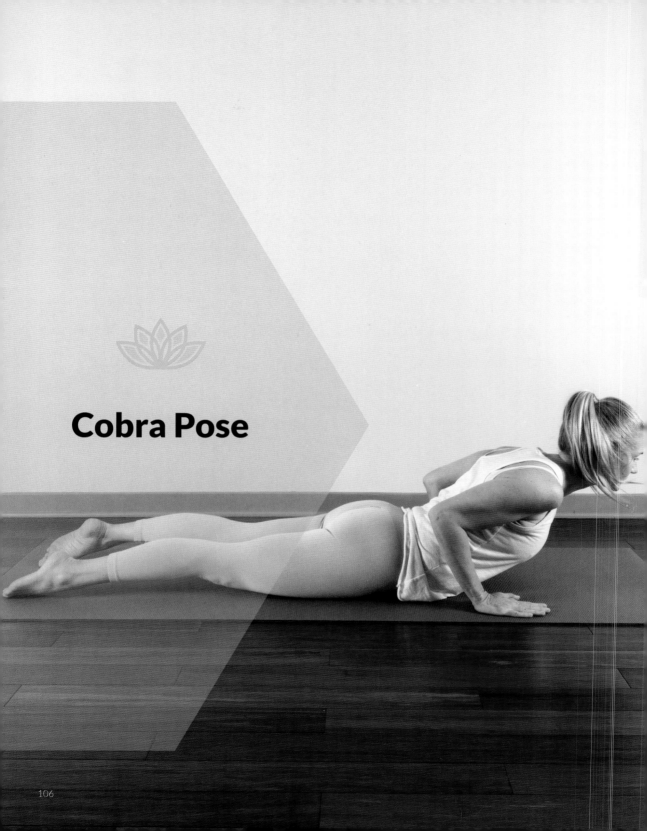

Cobra Pose

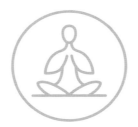

Cobra pose is a deeper variation than sphinx pose and strengthens your arms, shoulders and back. Begin by lying on your belly and resting your forehead on the mat. Keep your legs parallel and the tops of your feet down. Before you lift up, place your hands at the sides of your ribcage with bent elbows. Use your upper back muscles to lift you up as your elbows point behind you. Avoid straining your neck as you rise up. Keep your legs, feet and hip bones on the mat as you use your upper back muscles to lift you, rather than your hands or your neck.

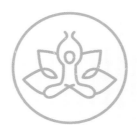

Gate Pose

Gate pose is a side stretch and gentle balance exercise. Start in a neutral kneeling position. Extend one leg to the side, resting your foot flat and slightly angled inward. Place your foot in line with your opposite knee. Lean away from your extended leg and rest your hand on the ground or on a block as pictured on page 110. Keep your hand directly underneath your shoulder.

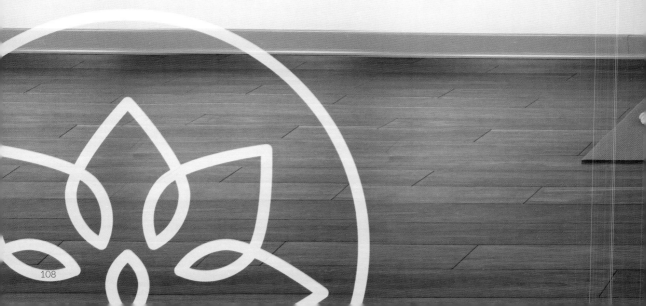

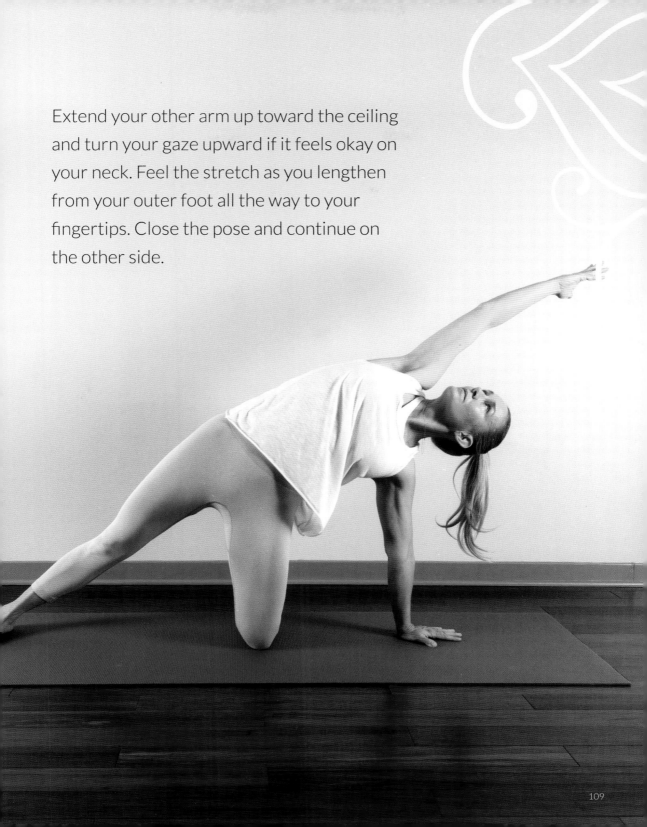

Extend your other arm up toward the ceiling and turn your gaze upward if it feels okay on your neck. Feel the stretch as you lengthen from your outer foot all the way to your fingertips. Close the pose and continue on the other side.

Gate Pose

Different levels of balance and even different lengths of arms and legs can affect gate pose. If the balance is too hard, use a block beneath your hand or even your back foot.

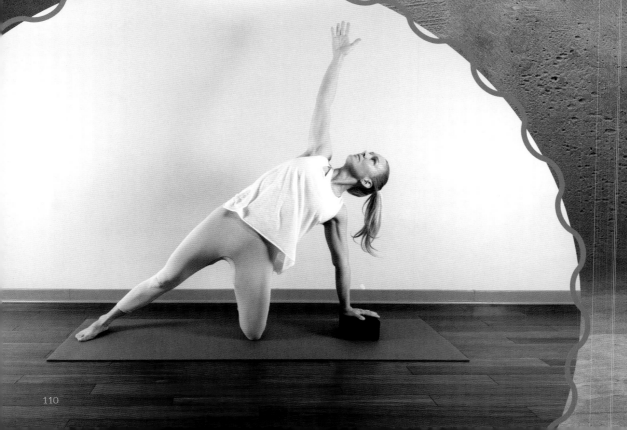

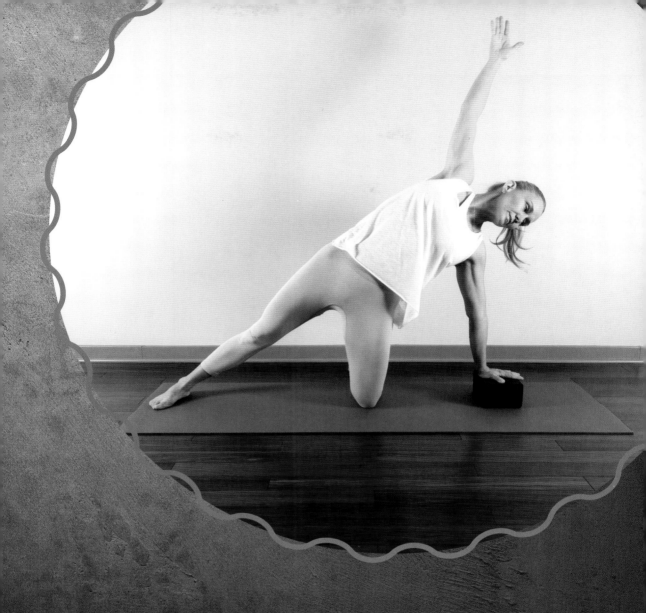

Bend your arm and rest it on your back as with rotated wide-legged forward fold. You can also let your head remain neutral, as seen above, rather than looking up toward your fingertips.

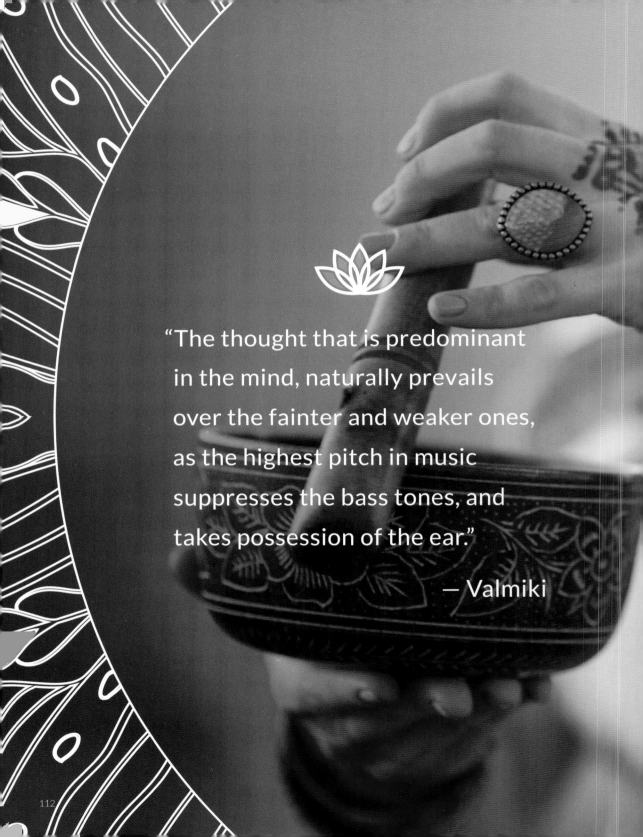

"The thought that is predominant in the mind, naturally prevails over the fainter and weaker ones, as the highest pitch in music suppresses the bass tones, and takes possession of the ear."

— Valmiki

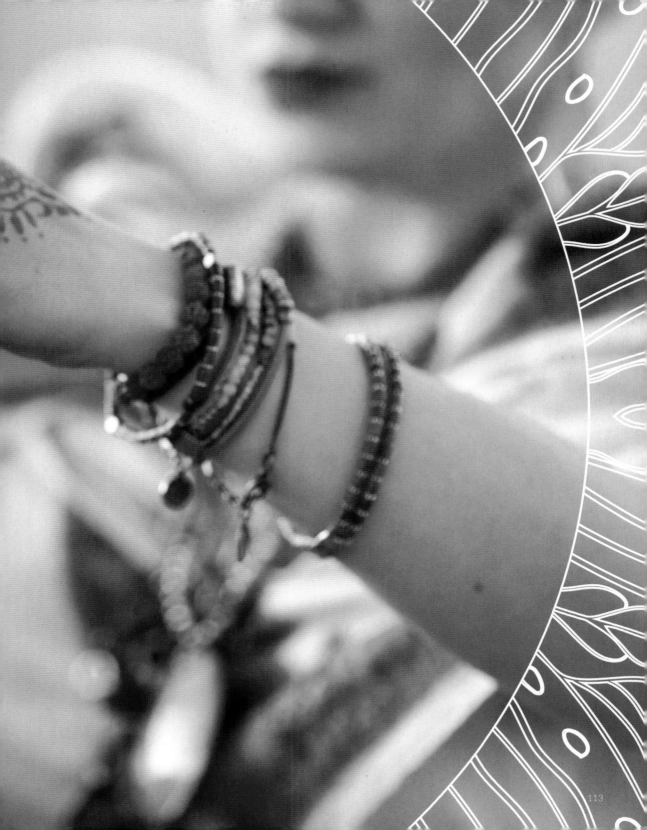

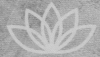

Low Lunge, 1

Low lunge pose releases tension in your hips and strengthens your leg muscles. Begin with table pose as you place one foot forward. Press the top of that foot into the mat along with the

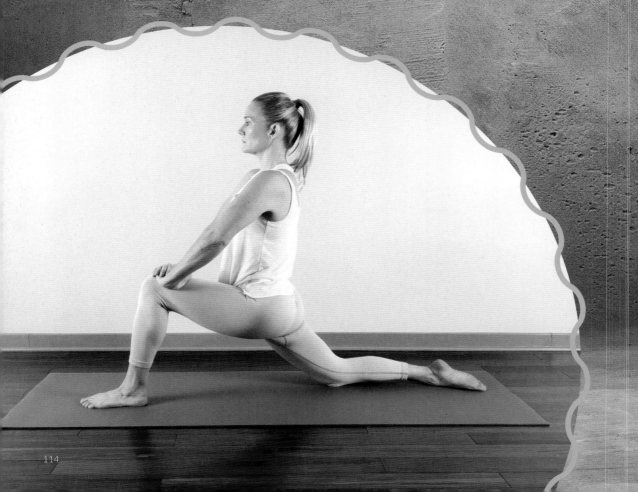

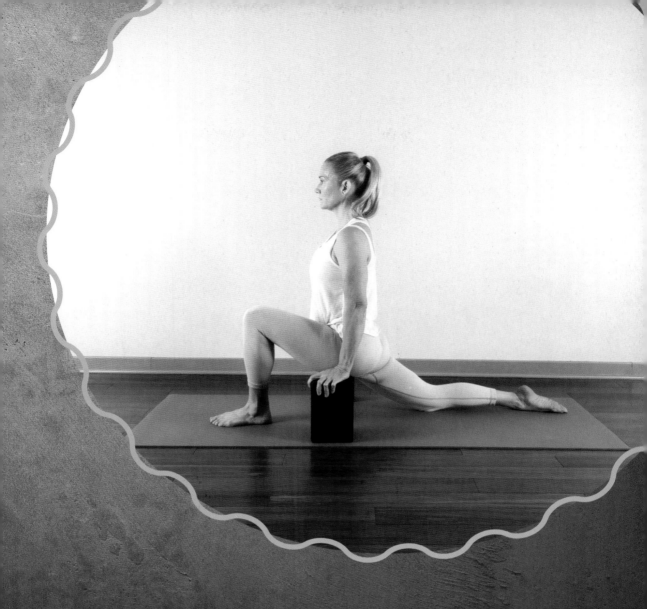

front of your back shin and top of your back foot. Keep your front knee directly over your front ankle. Place a blanket under your back knee if you have any discomfort.

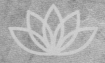

Half Splits

Half splits pose is an excellent complement to other forms of exercise, such as biking or running. From table pose, extend one leg in front of you, resting your heel on the floor but engaging the foot so your toes are pointing upward. Keep your hip aligned over your bent knee as you fold over your

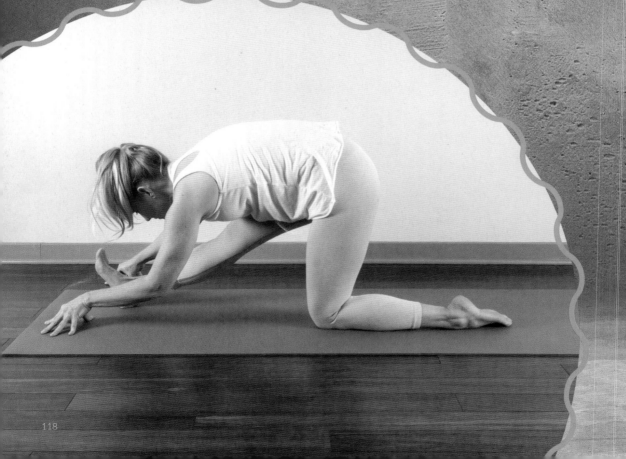

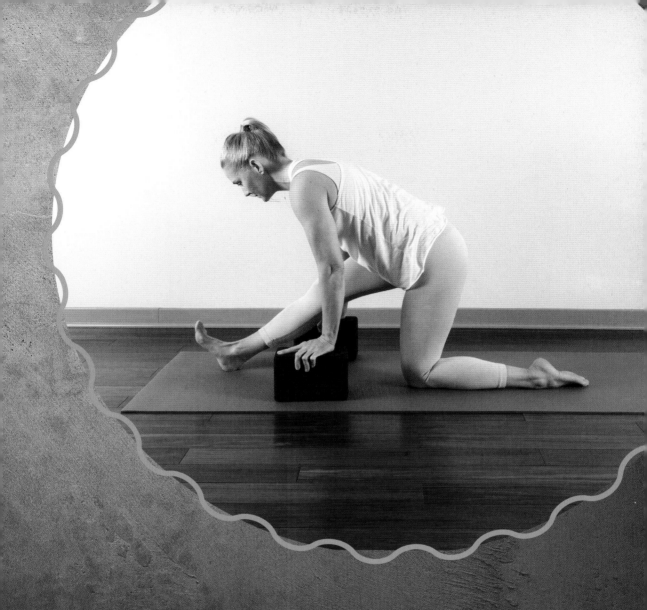

extended leg, reaching your nose toward your toes. You can use blocks to support your hands as you stretch, pictured above. Flexing your front foot will activate the stretch in your extended leg. Avoid collapsing over your extended leg as you reach your chest forward with a flat back. Breathe into the stretch and switch sides when ready.

Supine Poses

BRIDGE • WINDSHIELD WIPERS • RECLINING PIGEON • RECLINED SPINAL TWIST • HAPPY BABY • BALL POSE

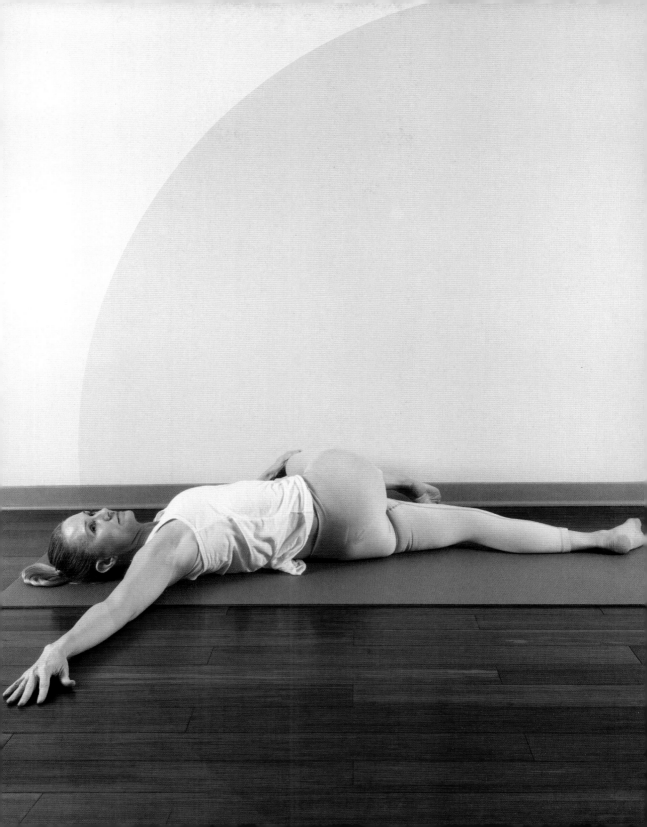

Bridge Pose

Bridge pose is a backbend that strengthens your legs and feet and opens your shoulders and hips. If you prefer a supported bridge pose, use a yoga block under your hips as pictured. Starting on your back, bend your knees and place your feet hips

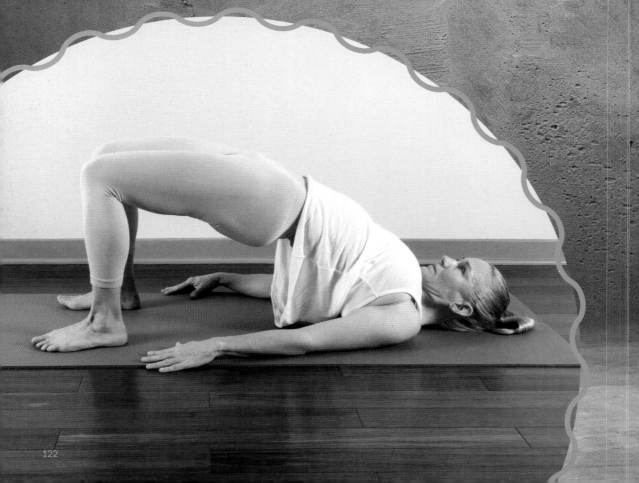

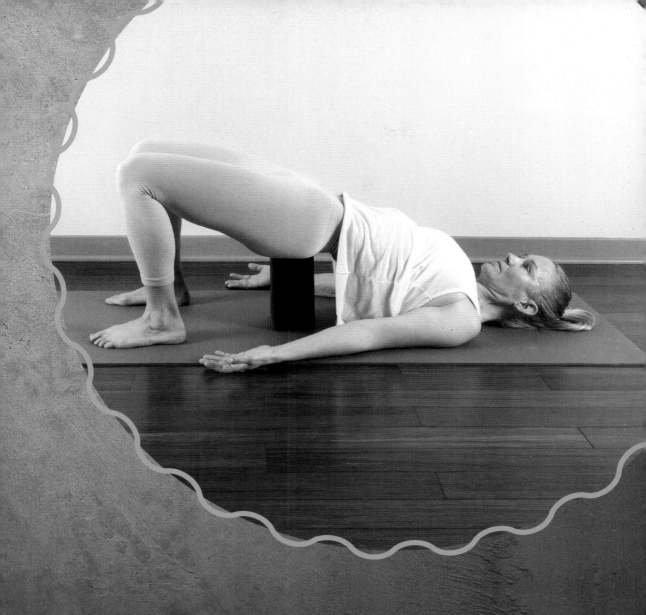

width and parallel on the floor. Stay
rooted through your feet as you lift
your hips, activating your inner
thighs to do so. Place the block

under your hips for support
(above), or clasp your hands under
your back to bring your shoulder
blades closer together.

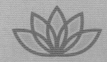

Windshield Wipers

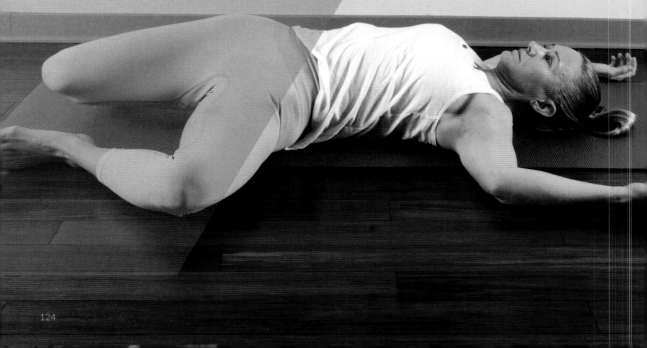

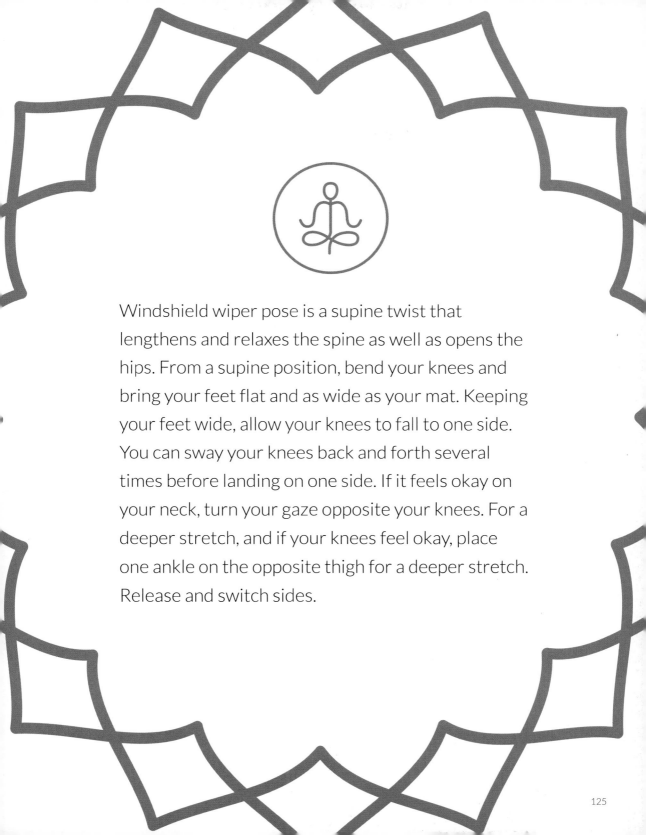

Windshield wiper pose is a supine twist that lengthens and relaxes the spine as well as opens the hips. From a supine position, bend your knees and bring your feet flat and as wide as your mat. Keeping your feet wide, allow your knees to fall to one side. You can sway your knees back and forth several times before landing on one side. If it feels okay on your neck, turn your gaze opposite your knees. For a deeper stretch, and if your knees feel okay, place one ankle on the opposite thigh for a deeper stretch. Release and switch sides.

Reclining Pigeon

Reclining pigeon pose is a deep hip stretch conducted from a prone position. Starting on your back, bend your knees and place your feet hips width and parallel on the floor. Lift one leg and rest the ankle on the thigh of your opposite leg, forming a triangle.

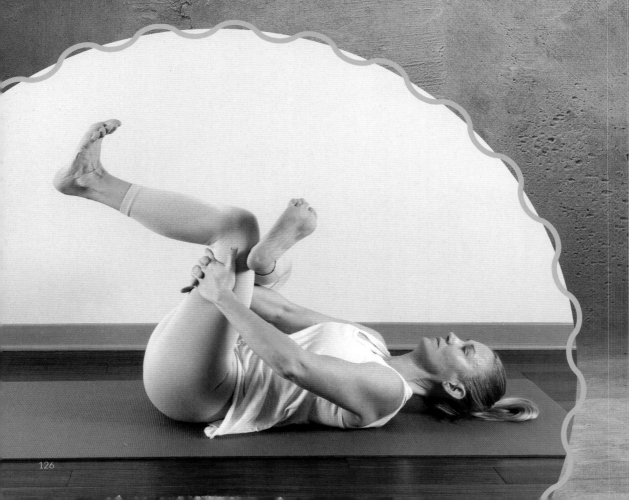

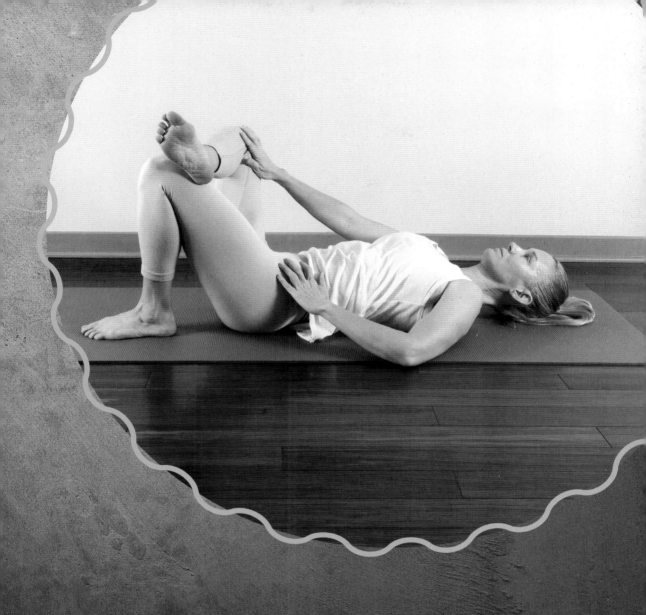

Clasp your hands around that thigh, or use a strap, and gently pull it toward your upper body as you bring your calf parallel to the floor. Flex your feet to feel more of the stretch in your hips and the back of your leg. Hold the pose and breathe, then release it, placing both feet back on the floor. Switch sides and repeat.

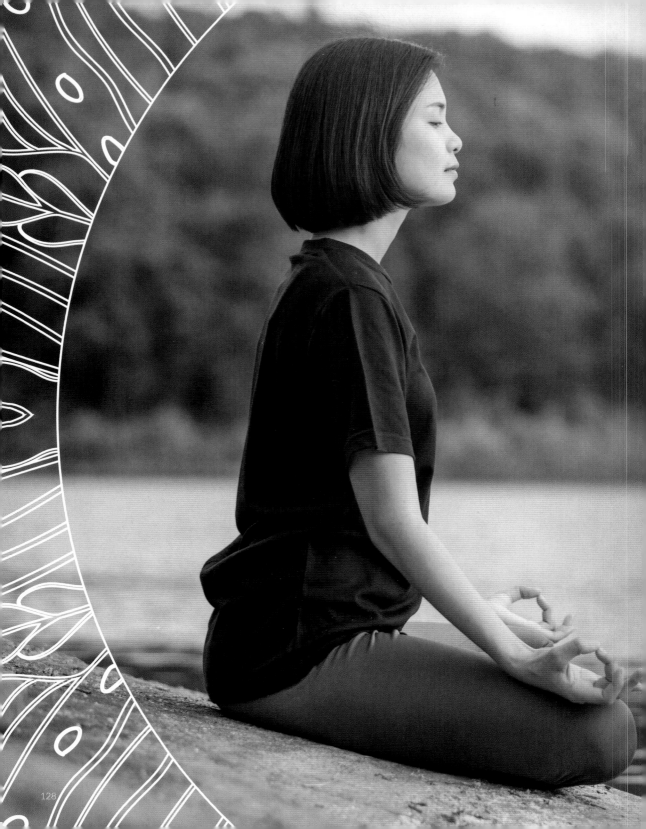

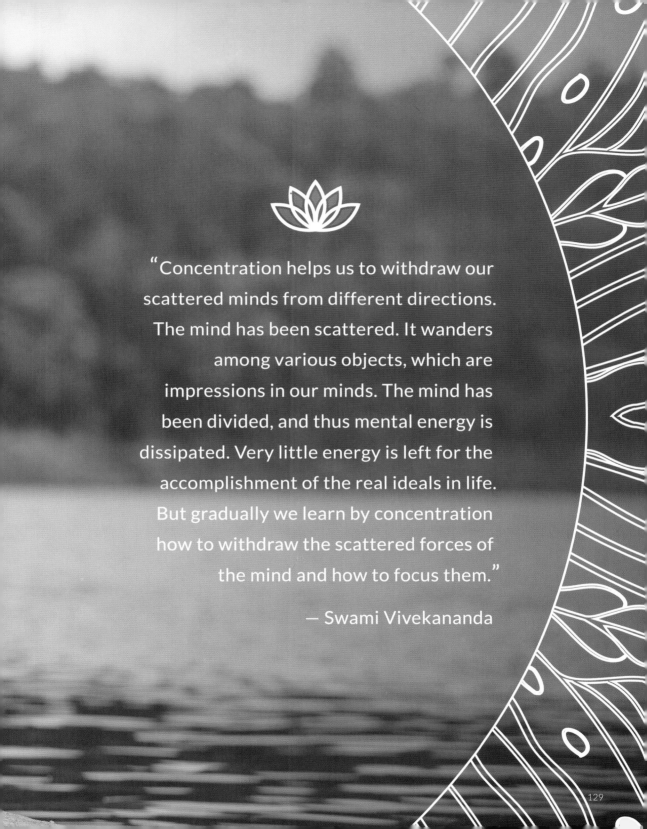

"Concentration helps us to withdraw our scattered minds from different directions. The mind has been scattered. It wanders among various objects, which are impressions in our minds. The mind has been divided, and thus mental energy is dissipated. Very little energy is left for the accomplishment of the real ideals in life. But gradually we learn by concentration how to withdraw the scattered forces of the mind and how to focus them."

— Swami Vivekananda

Reclined Spinal Twist

Reclined spinal twist lengthens and relaxes the spine from a prone position. Hug one knee into your chest as you extend your other leg long and flex the foot. Using the hand opposite your bent knee, clasp the knee as you extend the other arm out to

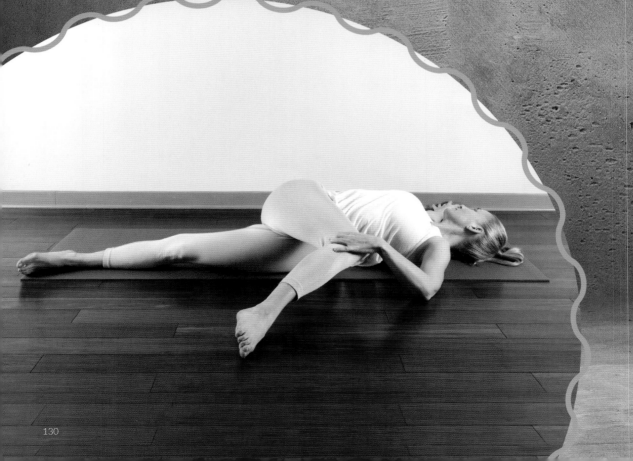

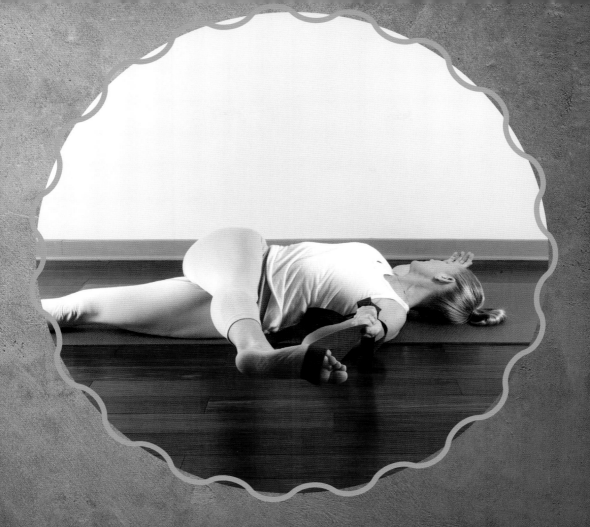

the side. Keep both shoulders on the floor as you bring your bent knee up and over, stacking one hip over the other. You'll feel your spine lengthen and stretch as well as your back and leg. Breathe in and out as you let your spine lengthen, then return to prone position and switch sides.

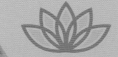

Knees to Chest Pose

Knees to chest pose is an excellent low back release and centering exercise. From a prone position, bring one hand to each knee or shin and hug your knees to your chest. Practice rocking side to side as your massage your low back into the mat. You may also practice bringing your nose up to your knees as you activate your core to lift you, being careful not to strain your neck. Create more movement by resting your head on the mat and taking circles with your knees to massage your low back or separate your knees and circle them to massage your hip joints.

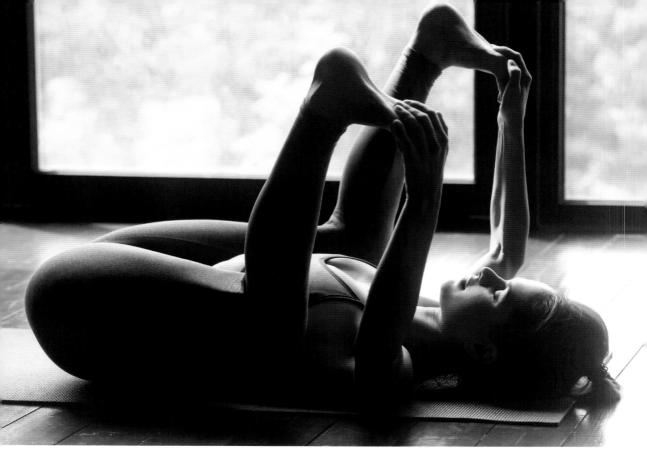

Happy Baby

Happy baby pose is a hip and thigh stretch, as well as a low back release. Start with knees to chest pose and then separate and flex your feet toward the ceiling. Clasp your outer feet, ankles or thighs as you bring your knees toward your armpits. If it is challenging to hold your feet, you can use a strap, as

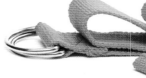

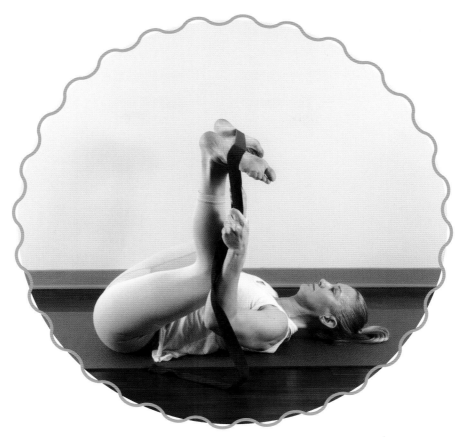

pictured. You may also rest your head on a yoga block or blanket to avoid straining your neck. Feel your hips open and your low back release as you take several inhales and exhales.

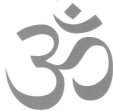

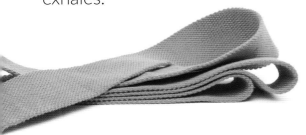

meditation.
breath.
fitness.

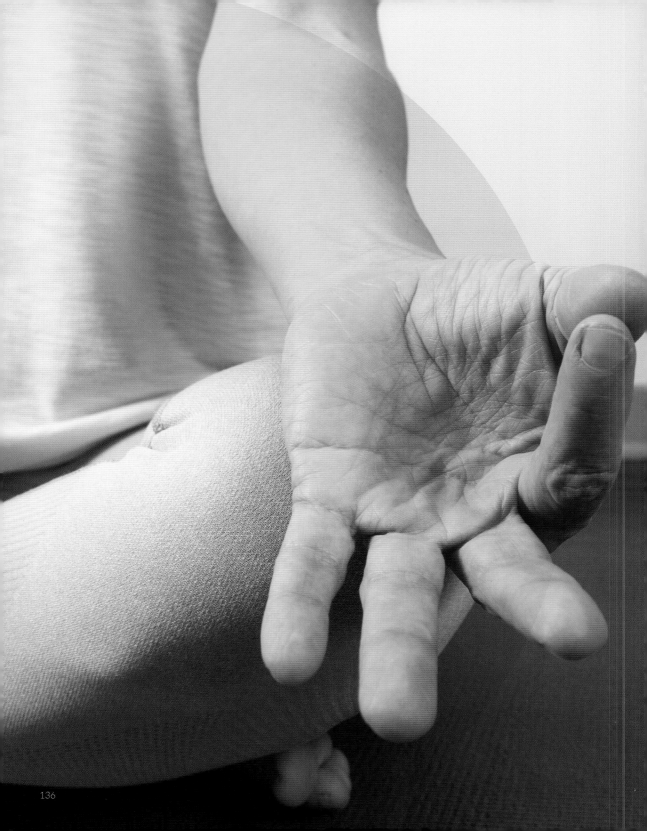

Closing Poses

CORPSE POSE • LEGS UP THE WALL •
SEATED ANJALI HANDS

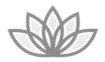

Corpse Pose

Corpse pose, or **savasana**, is a resting pose to be taken at the end of every yoga practice. Lie on your back with your legs comfortable, your arms resting wide at your sides and palms facing up. Relax your muscles and feel

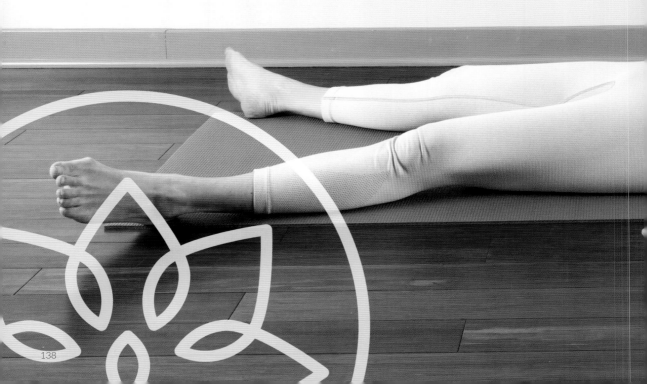

your body "melt" into the mat as you close your eyes and breathe. If it is uncomfortable to lie straight on your back, you can place a rolled up blanket or cushion under your knees. This position is typically practiced for at least five minutes as you breathe and let go.

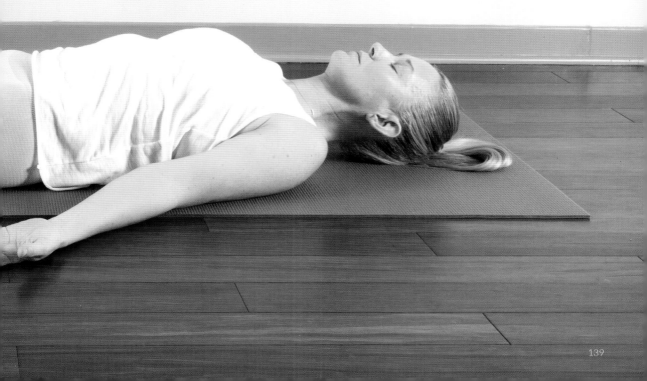

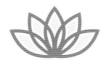

Legs Up the Wall

Legs up the wall pose is a restorative posture that allows the mind to relax as you breathe and relieve tension in the body. It's often used as the last or almost last pose in a sequence. From a seated position, bring one hip to the wall as you reach your legs up and around to achieve the position shown.

You may need to use your hands and arms to assist you into the position. Your hips and legs may be flush with the wall as shown on these pages, or they may angle slightly away. Either way produces an excellent relaxation benefit. It is recommended to stay in this position for at least five minutes as you breathe and let go.

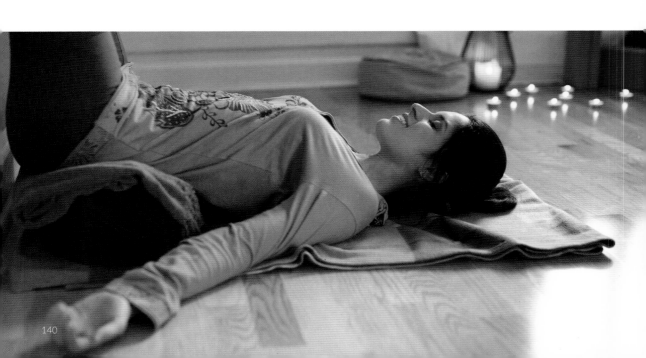

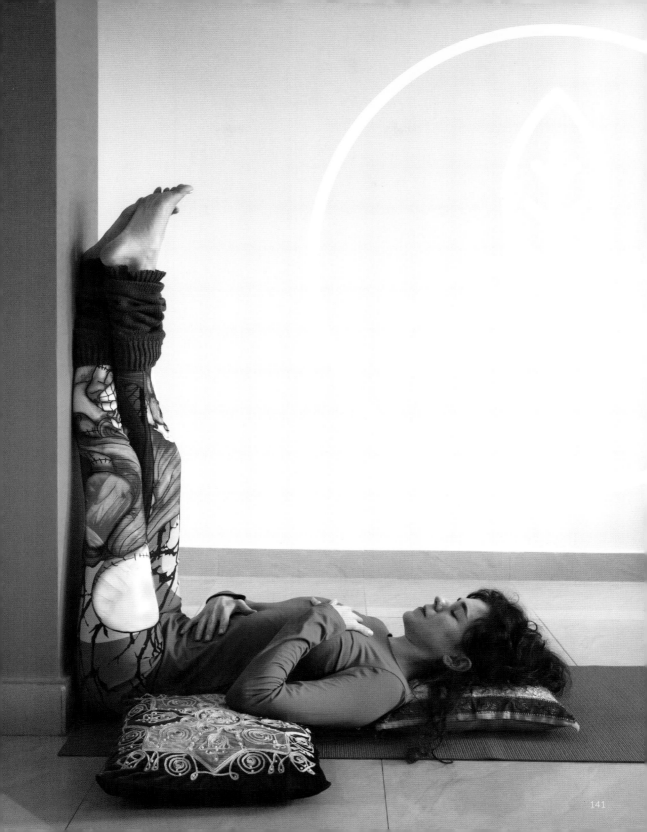

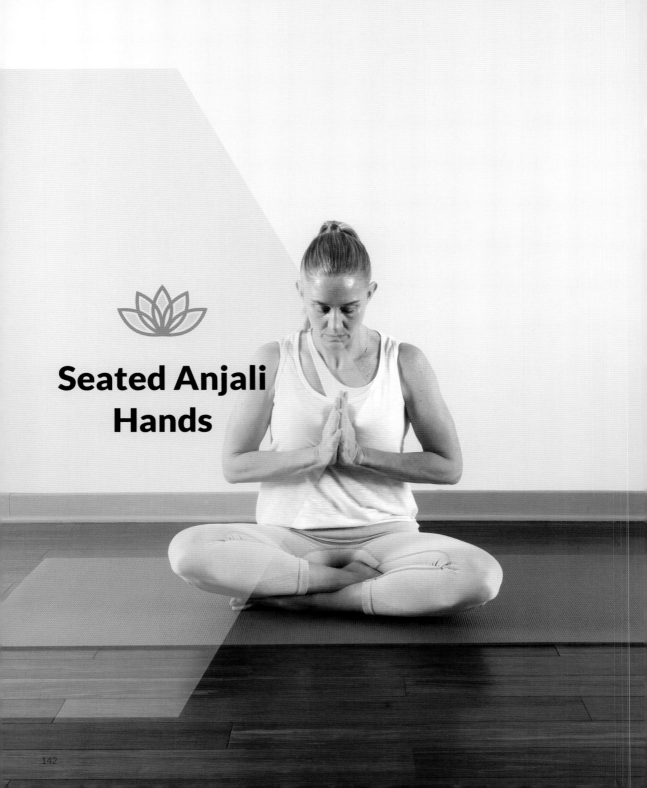

Seated Anjali Hands

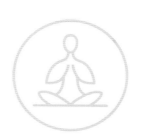

Seated pose often reappears at the end of a sequence as a way to focus energy and reflect on the sequence just completed. Sit with your legs crossed, using folded blankets or a yoga block to lift your hips if you need them, or sit on a firm cushion like a bolster. Lengthen your spine as you bring your shoulders up toward your ears and then roll them down your back, bringing your shoulder blades closer together. Feel your chest lift. Reach the the top of your head toward the ceiling as your spine lengthens. Bring your hands together at the center of your chest as you take long, slow inhales and exhales.

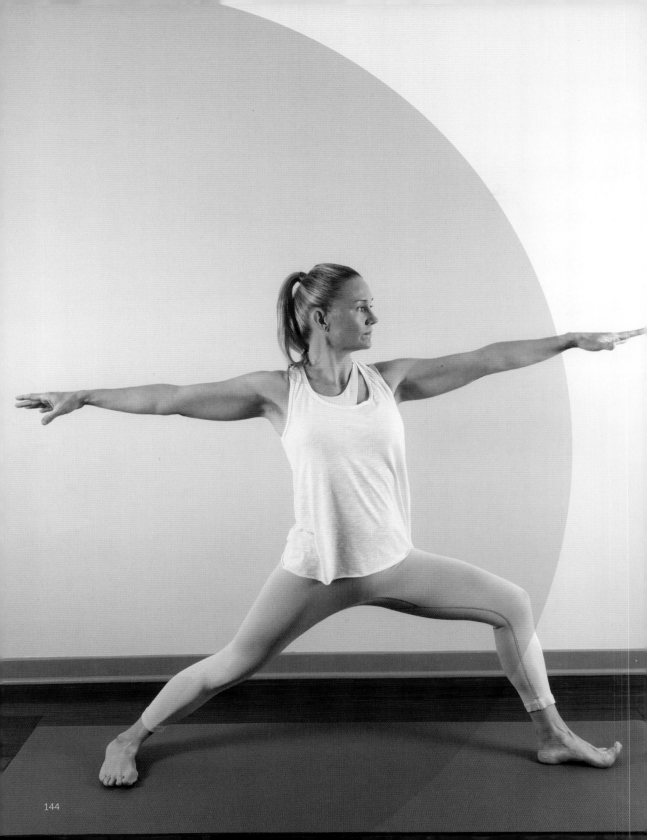

Sequences

30-MINUTE MAT SEQUENCE

45-MINUTE STANDING SEQUENCE

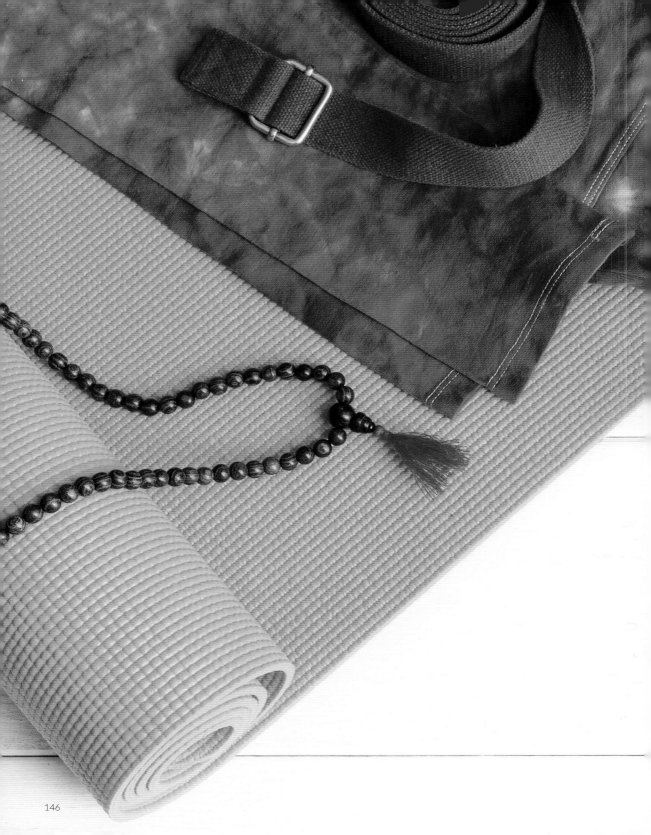

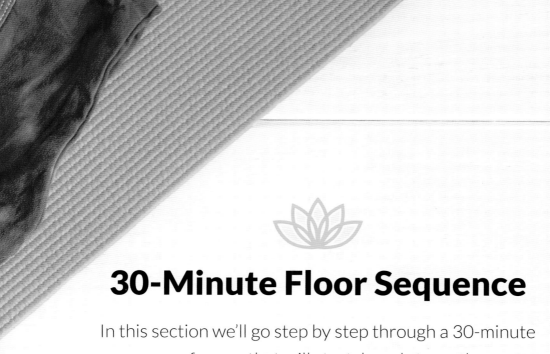

30-Minute Floor Sequence

In this section we'll go step by step through a 30-minute sequence of poses that will stretch and strengthen your body with gentle but effective motions.

1. Seated Pose
2. Neck Rolls
3. Seated Twist
4. Seated Side Stretch
5. Butterfly Pose
6. Table to Cat & Cow
7. Table to Spinal Balance
8. Table to Puppy Pose
9. Sphynx Pose
10. Child's Pose
11. Downward Facing Dog
12. Staff Pose
13. Head to Knee Pose
14. Seated Forward Fold
15. Bridge Pose
16. Windshield Wiper Pose
17. Happy Baby
18. Corpse Pose

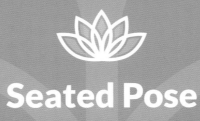

Seated Pose

Breathe in and out for 3 to 5 minutes.

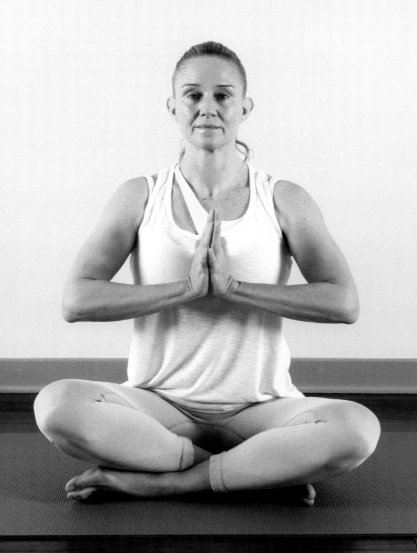

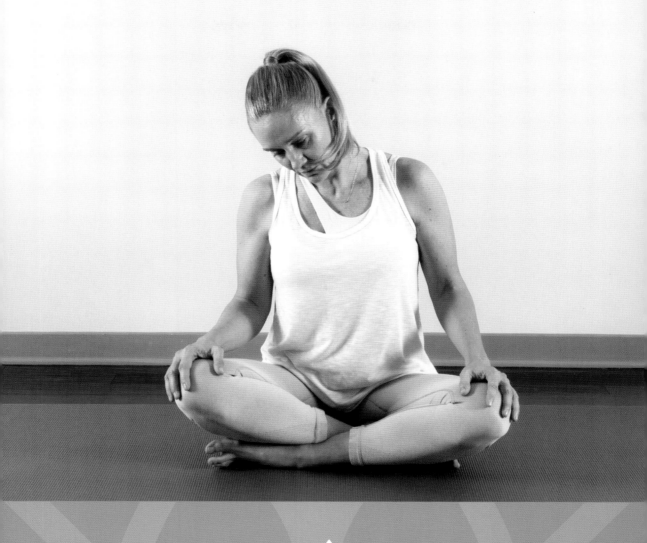

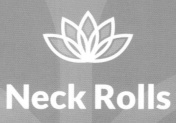

Neck Rolls

Roll 4 or 5 times in each direction.

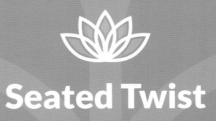

Seated Twist

Hold each side for 3 to 5 full exhales and inhales.

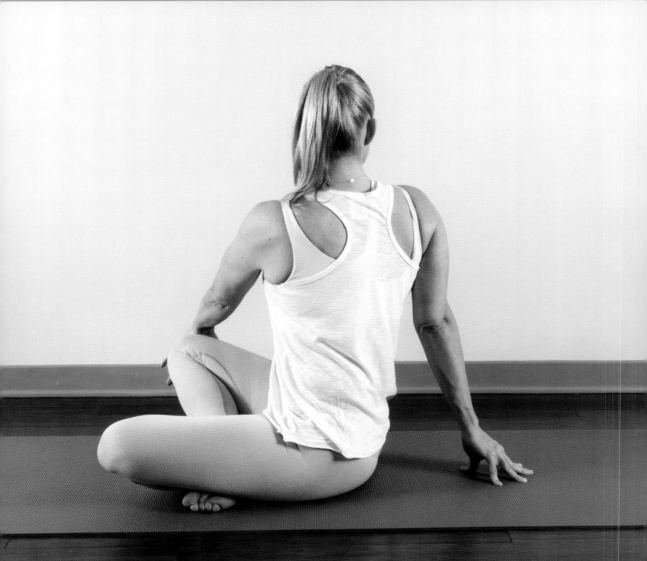

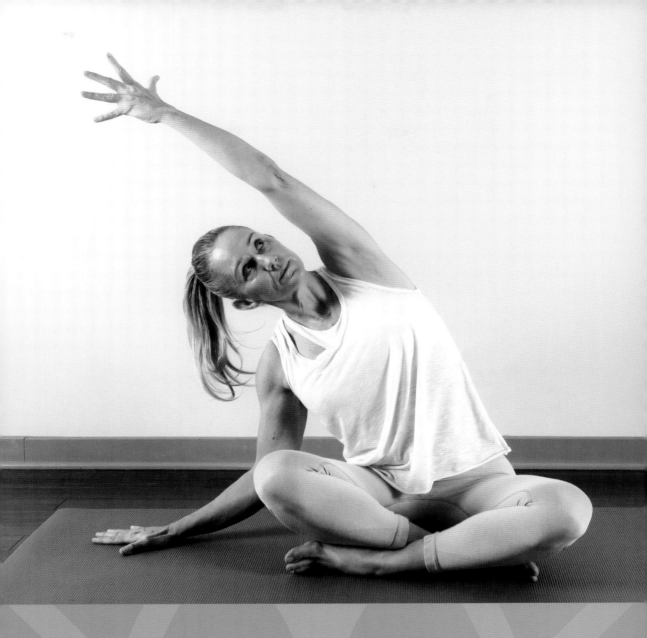

Seated Side Stretch

Hold each side for 3 to 5 full exhales and inhales.

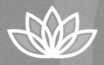

Butterfly Pose

Hold for 5 full exhales and inhales.

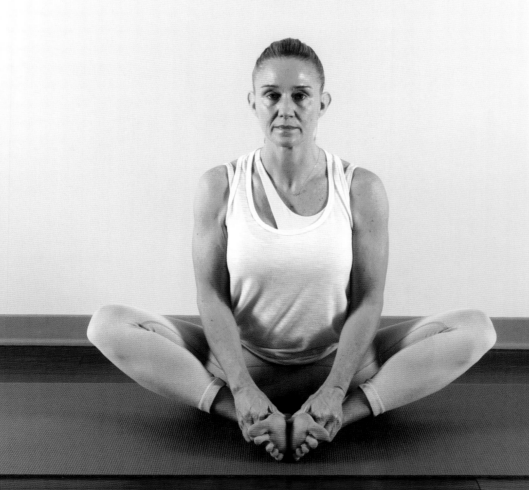

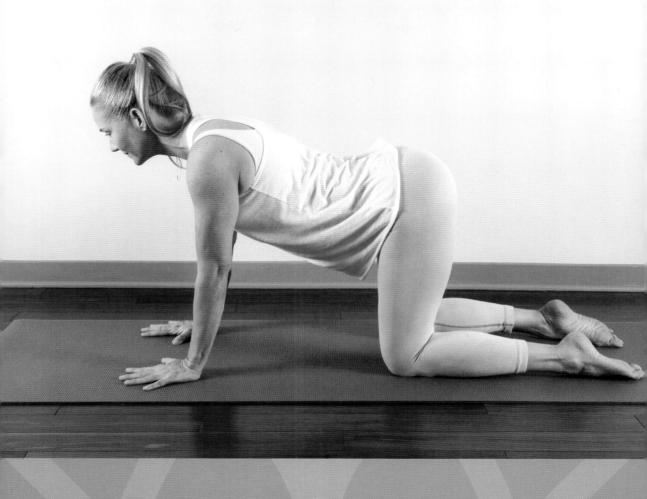

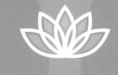

Table, Cat, & Cow

Begin in table pose, bowing into cow pose and
arching into cat pose for 8 to 10 full cycles.

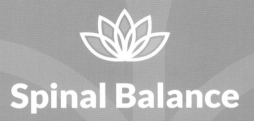

Spinal Balance

Begin in table pose. Raise alternating arms and legs,
holding each side for 3 full inhales and exhales.

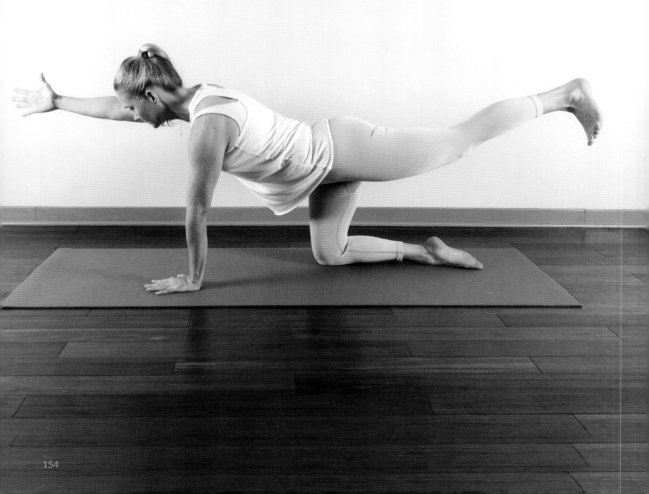

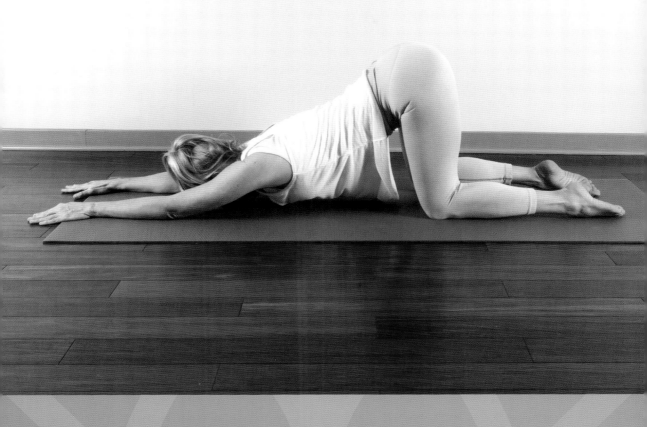

Puppy Pose

Begin in table pose. Move to puppy pose and
hold for 3 full inhales and exhales.

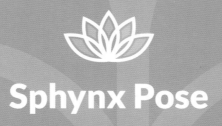

Sphynx Pose

Hold for 3 to 5 full inhales and exhales.

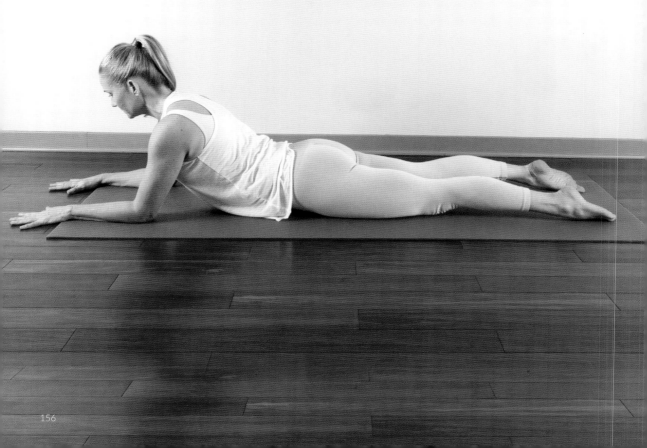

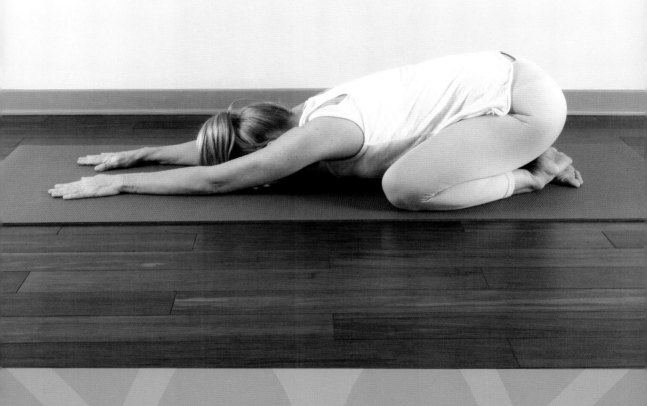

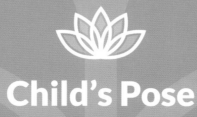

Child's Pose

Choose child pose with arms at your sides or active child
pose seen above. Hold for 5 full inhales and exhales.

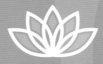

Downward Facing Dog

Hold for 5 full inhales and exhales.

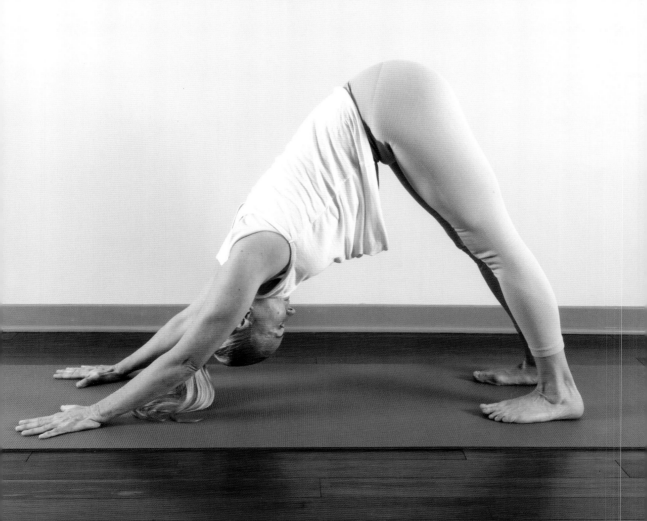

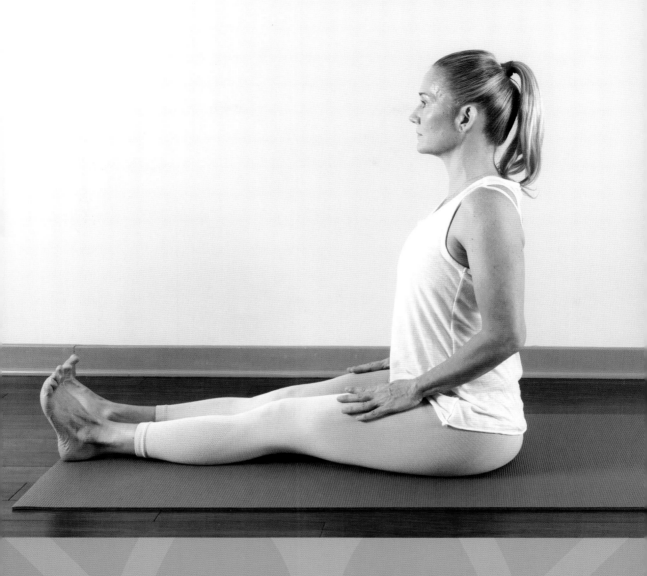

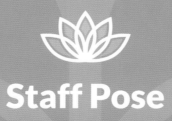

Staff Pose

Hold for 3 to 5 full inhales and exhales.

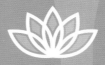

Head to Knee Pose

Hold each side for 5 full inhales and exhales.

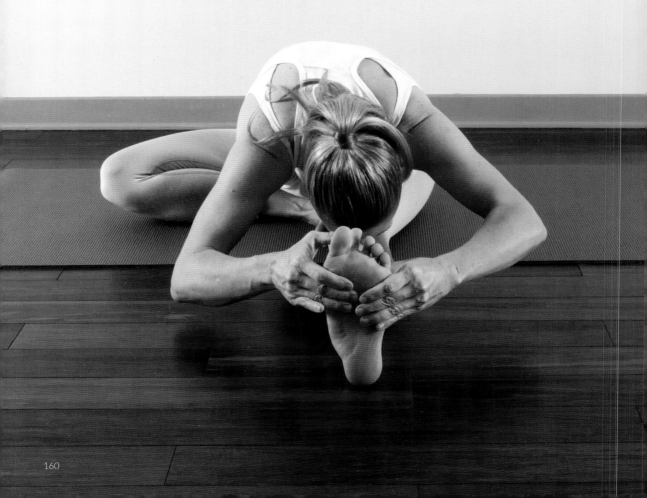

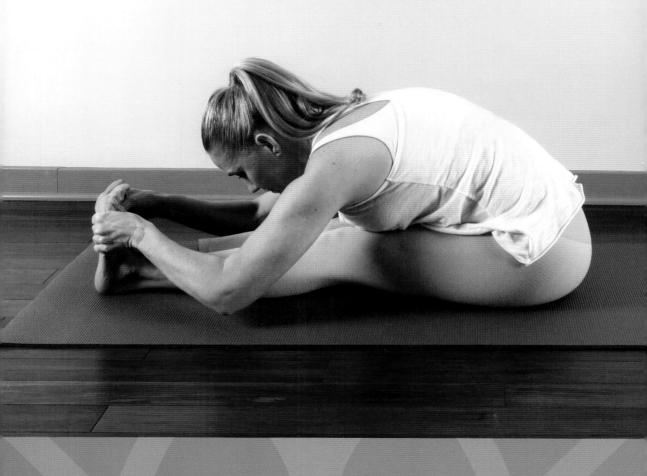

Seated Forward Fold

Hold for 5 full inhales and exhales.

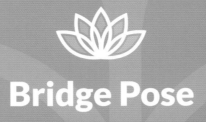

Bridge Pose

Hold for 5 full inhales and exhales.

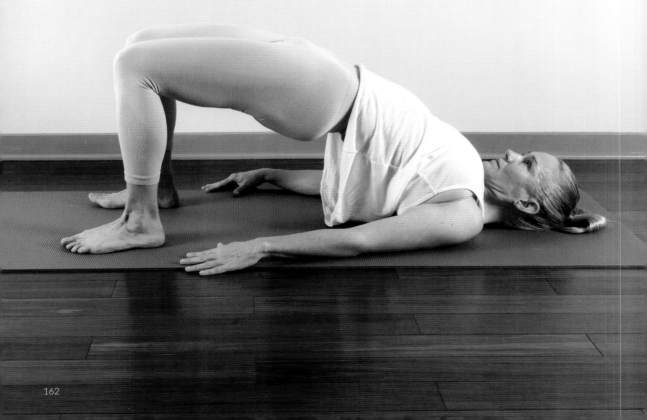

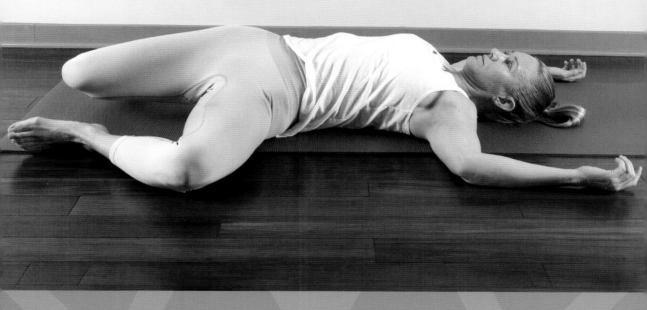

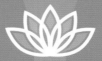

Windshield Wiper Pose

Hold each side for 3 to 5 full inhales and exhales.

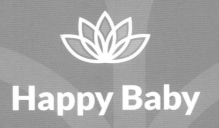

Happy Baby

Hold for 5 full inhales and exhales.

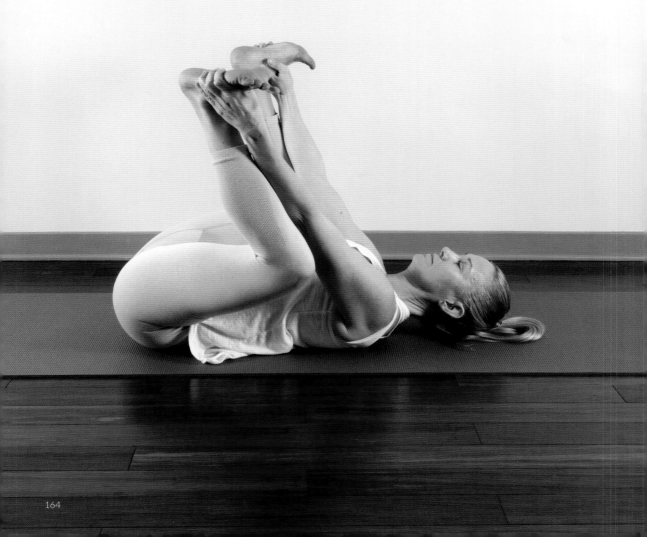

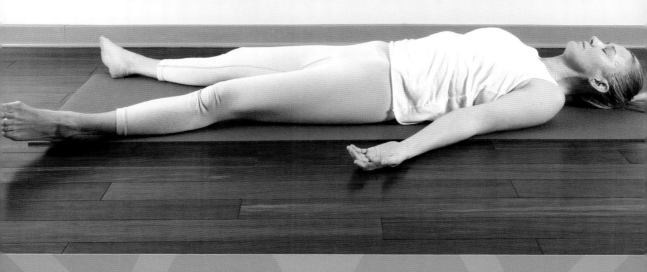

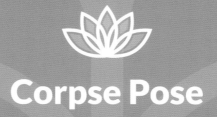

Corpse Pose

Hold for 5 minutes, letting yourself relax and melt further and further into the mat.

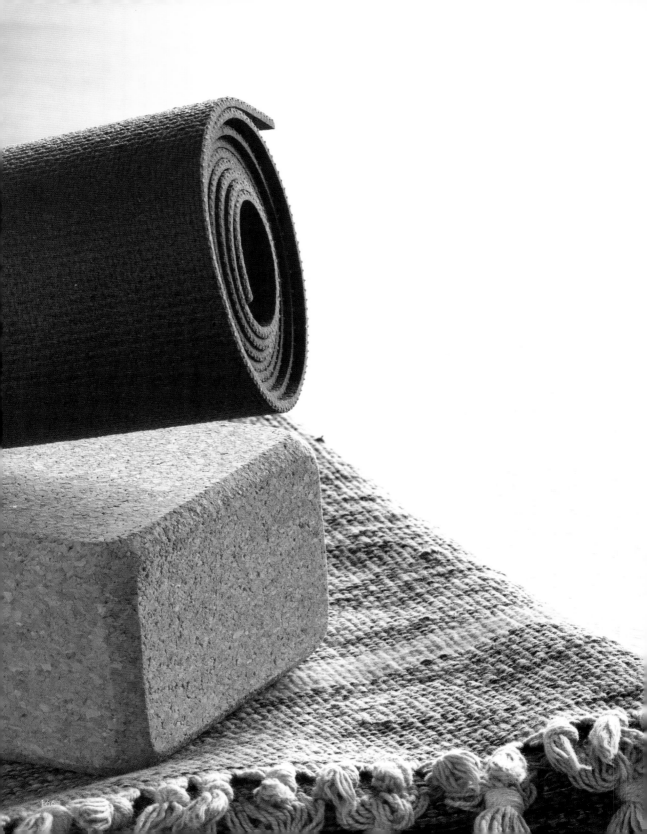

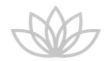

45-Minute Standing Sequence

In this section we'll go step by step through a 45-minute sequence of poses that will stretch and strengthen your body with gentle but effective motions.

1. Mountain Pose
2. Half Sun Salutation
3. Warrior 2 Pose
4. Reverse Warrior
5. Triangle Pose
6. Extended Side Angle
7. Repeat 3–6
8. Wide Legged Forward Fold
9. Mountain Pose
10. Tree Pose
11. Standing Forward Fold
12. Table to Cat & Cow Pose
13. Low Lunge
14. Child's Pose
15. Downward Facing Dog
16. Staff Pose
17. Seated Forward Fold
18. Reclined Pigeon
19. Bridge Pose
20. Reclined Spinal Twist
21. Happy Baby
22. Corpse Pose

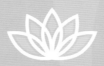

Mountain Pose

Hold for 3 minutes.

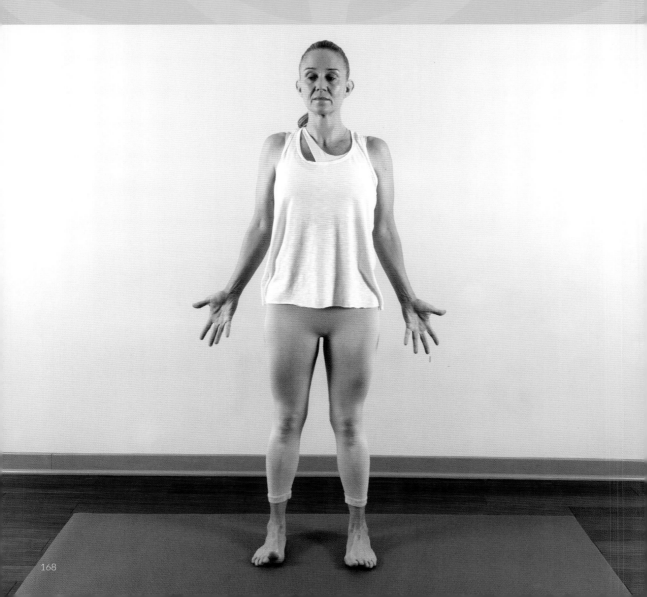

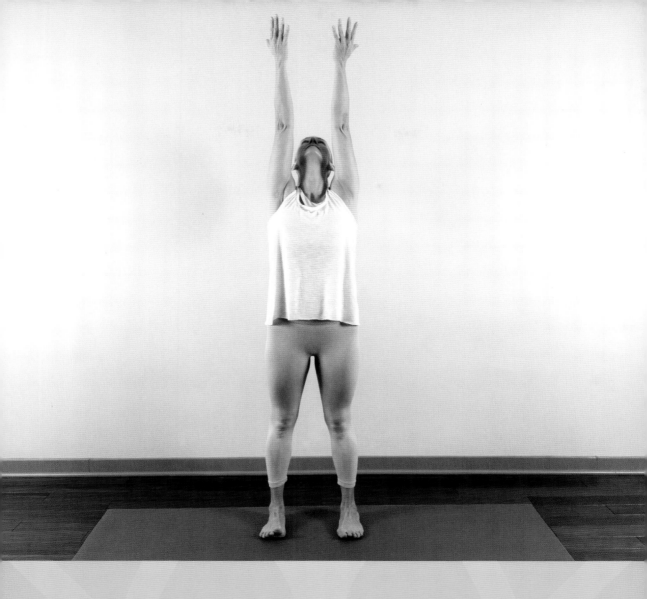

Half Sun Salutation

Flow through this salutation 5 times.

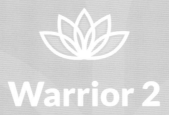

Warrior 2

Hold for 3 to 5 full inhales and exhales. For now, just do one side.

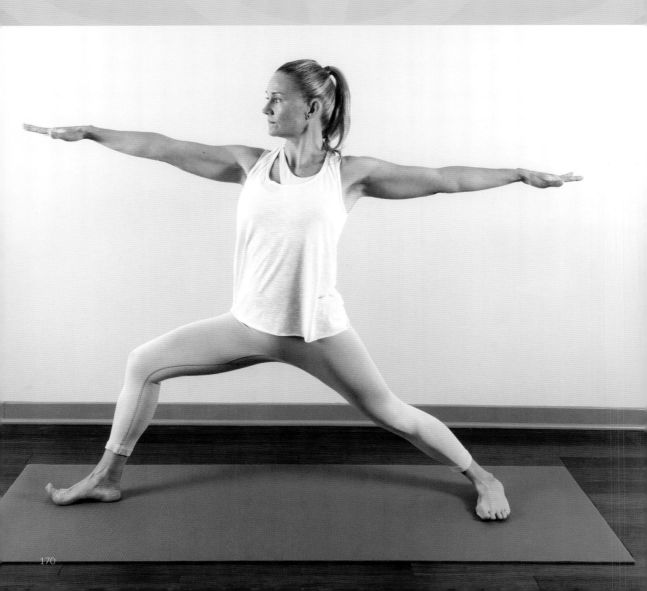

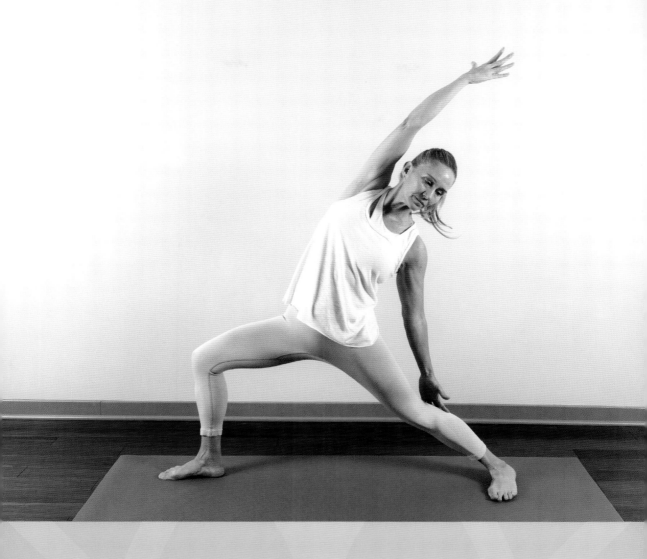

Reverse Warrior

Hold for 3 to 5 full inhales and exhales. For now, just do one side.

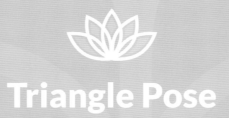

Triangle Pose

Hold for 3 to 5 full inhales and exhales. For now, just do one side.

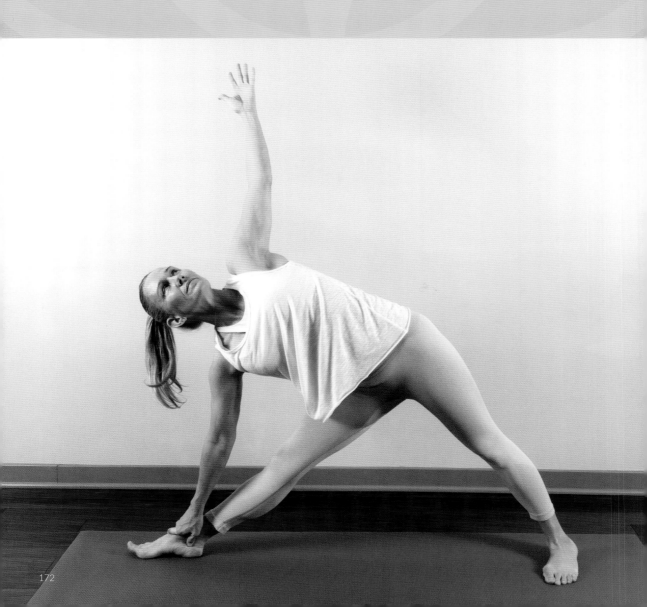

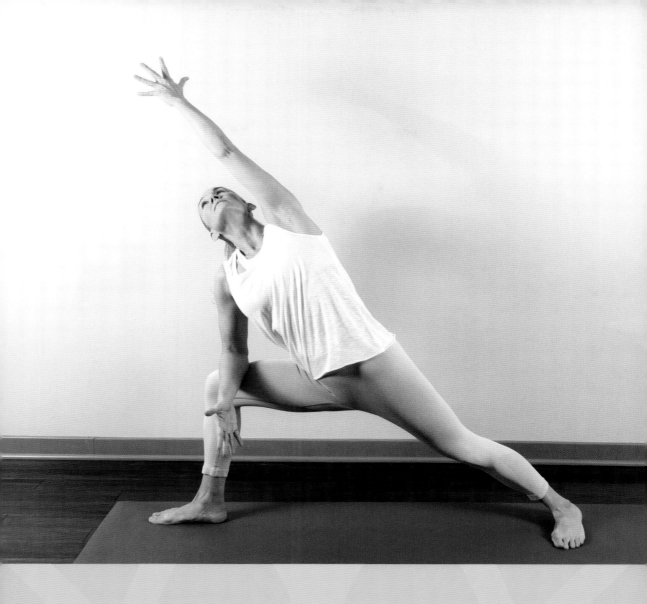

Extended Side Angle

Hold for 3 to 5 full inhales and exhales. For now, just do one side.

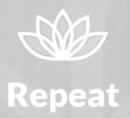

Repeat

Switch sides and repeat Warrior 2, Reverse Warrior,
Triangle Pose, and Extended Side Angle.

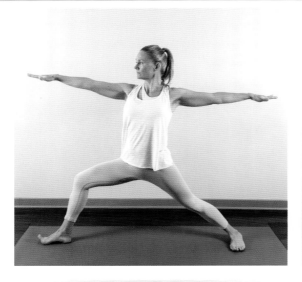

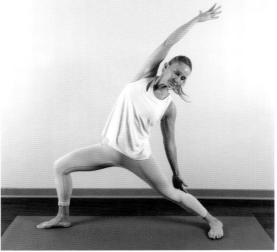

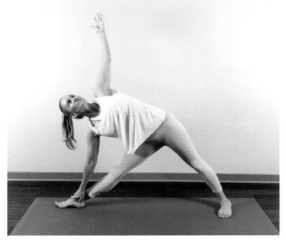

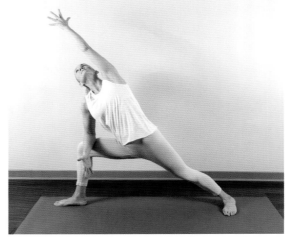

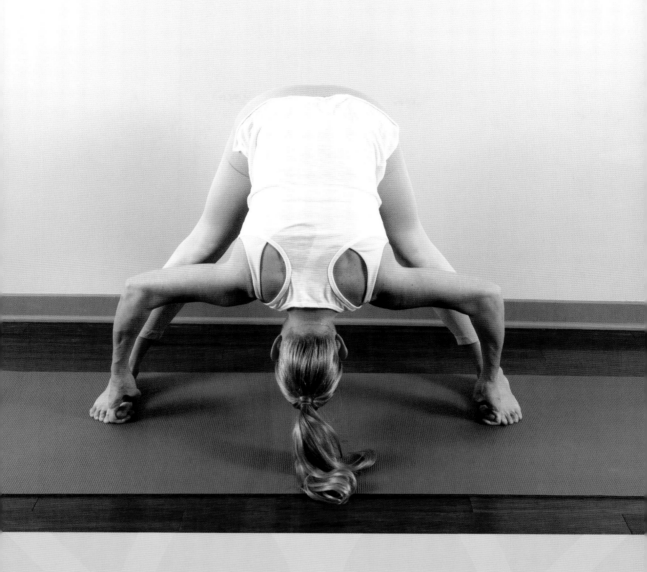

Wide Legged Forward Fold

Hold for 3 to 5 full inhales and exhales.

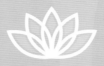

Mountain Pose

Hold for 3 to 5 full inhales and exhales.

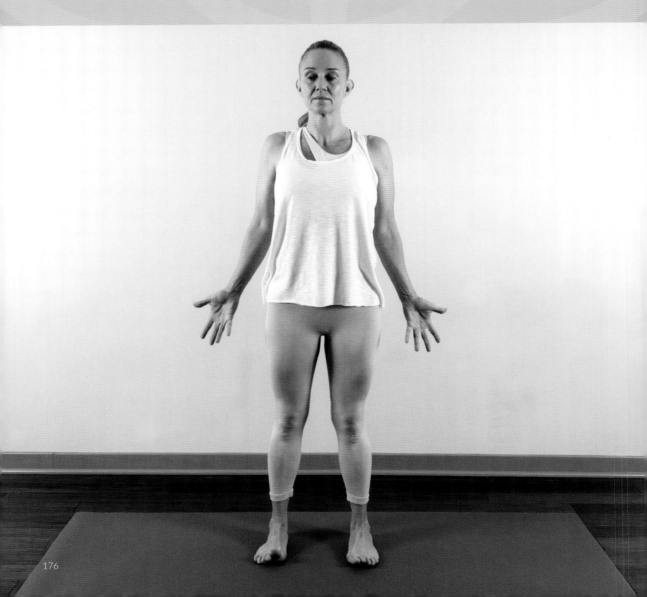

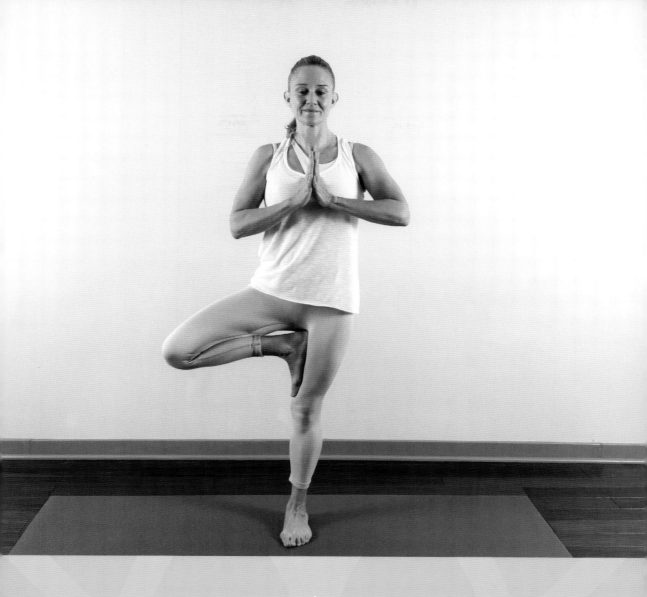

Tree Pose

Hold for 1 to 3 full inhales and exhales per side.

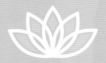

Standing Forward Fold

Hold for 3 to 5 full inhales and exhales.

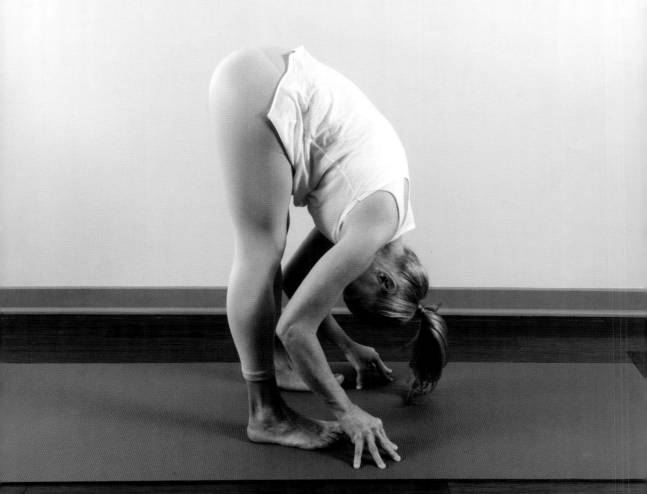

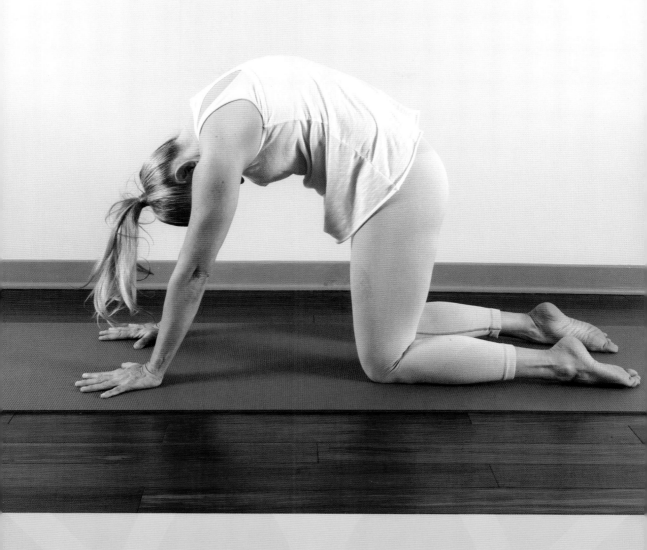

Table, Cat, & Cow

Begin in table pose and complete 8 to 10 full cycles of
bowing into cow pose and arching into cat pose.

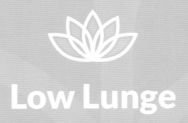

Low Lunge

Hold for 3 full inhales and exhales per side.

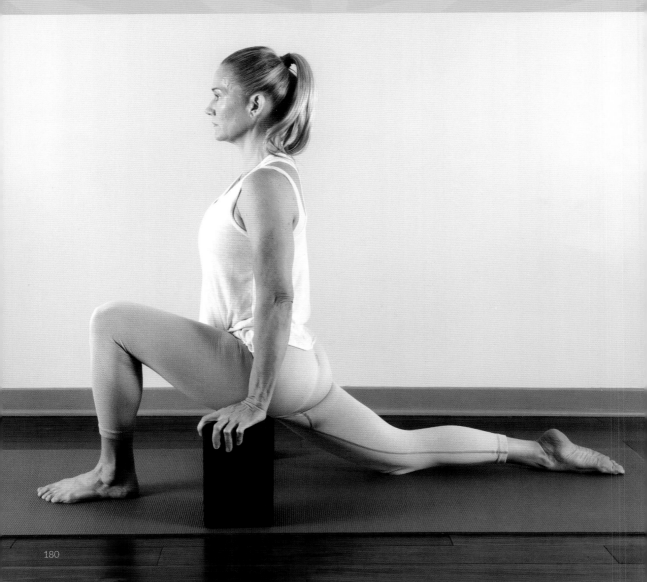

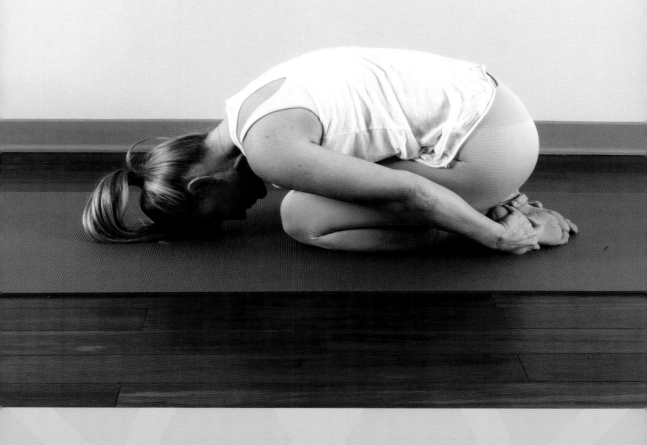

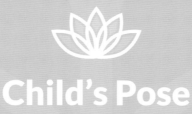

Child's Pose

Hold for 5 full inhales and exhales.

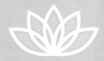

Downward Facing Dog

Hold for 5 full inhales and exhales.

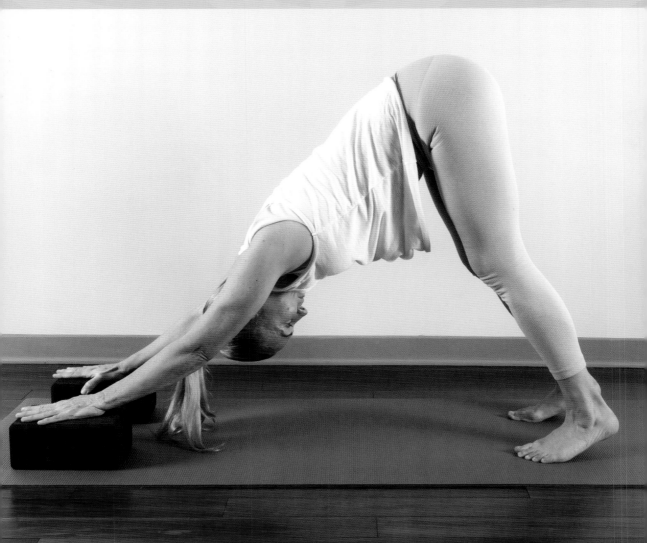

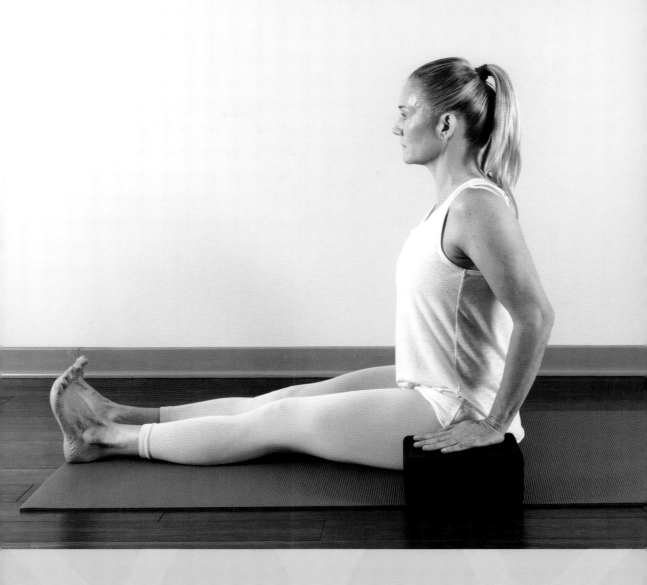

Staff Pose

Hold for 3 to 5 full inhales and exhales.

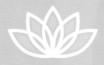

Seated Forward Fold

Hold for 5 full inhales and exhales.

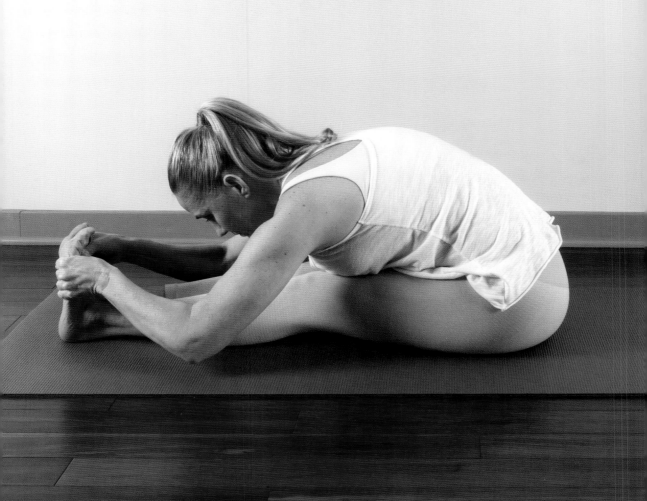

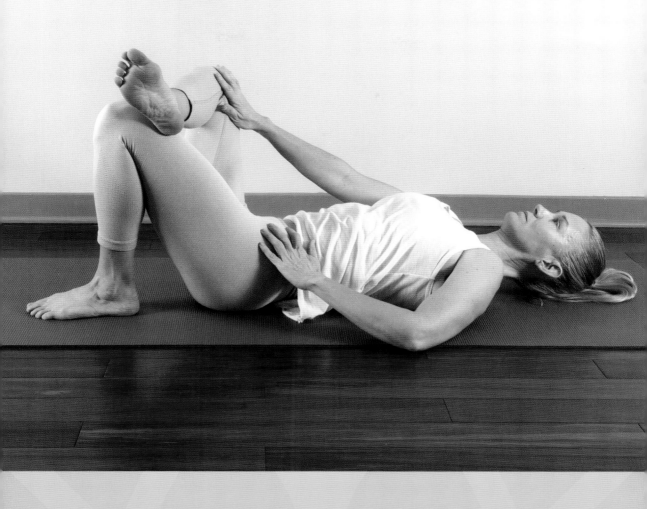

Reclined Pigeon

Hold for 3 to 5 full inhales and exhales per side.

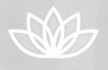

Bridge Pose

Hold for 5 full inhales and exhales.

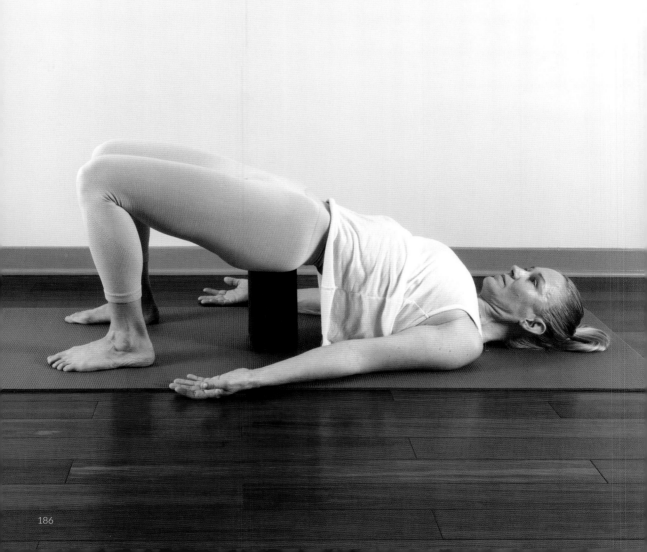

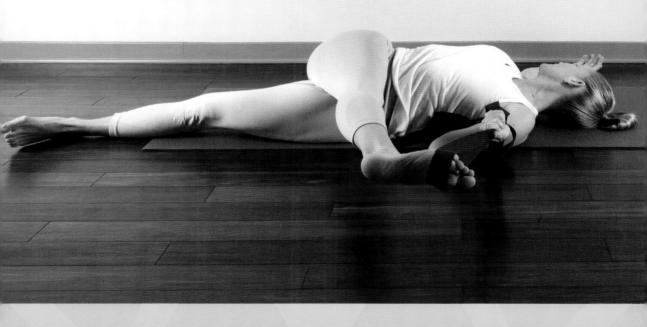

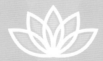

Reclined Spinal Twist

Hold for 5 full inhales and exhales per side.

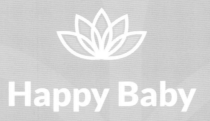

Happy Baby

Hold for 5 full inhales and exhales.

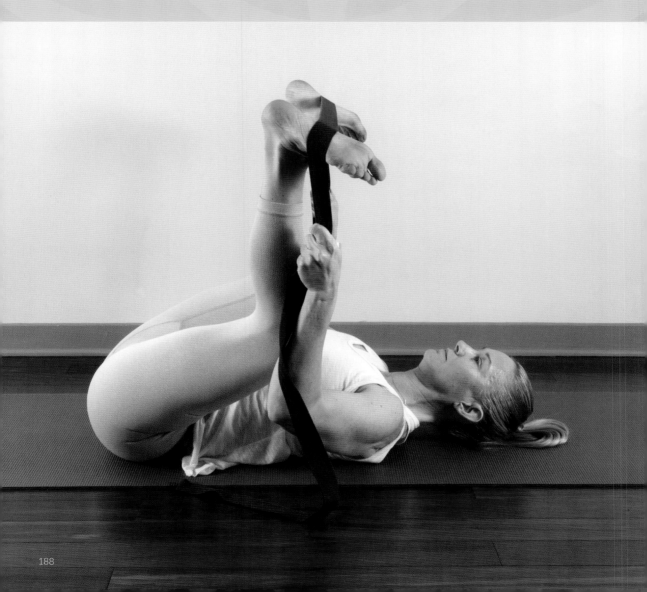

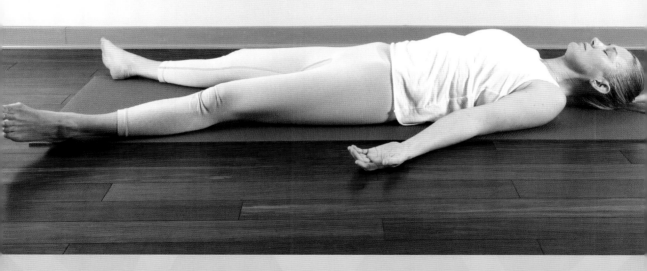

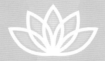

Corpse Pose

Hold for 5 minutes, allowing your body
to relax and melt into the mat.

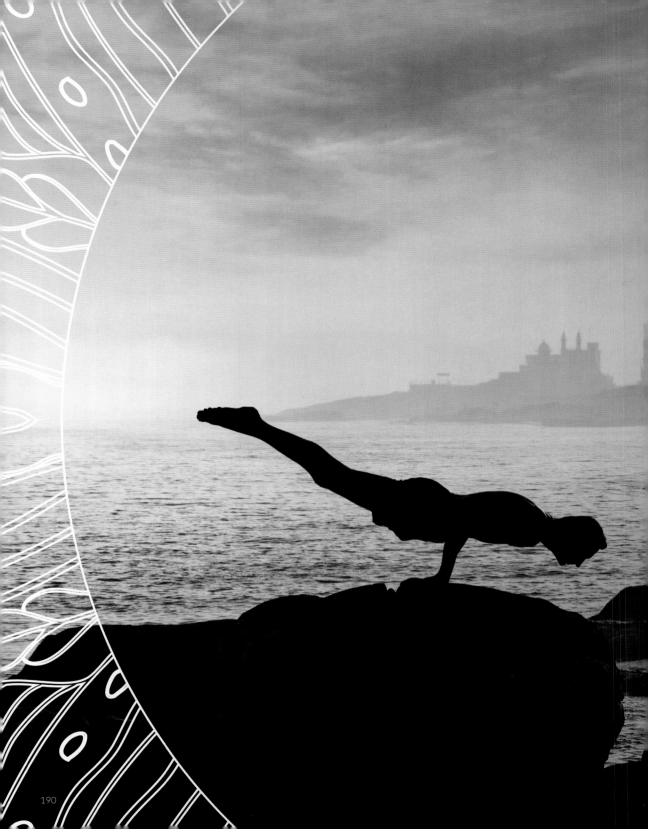

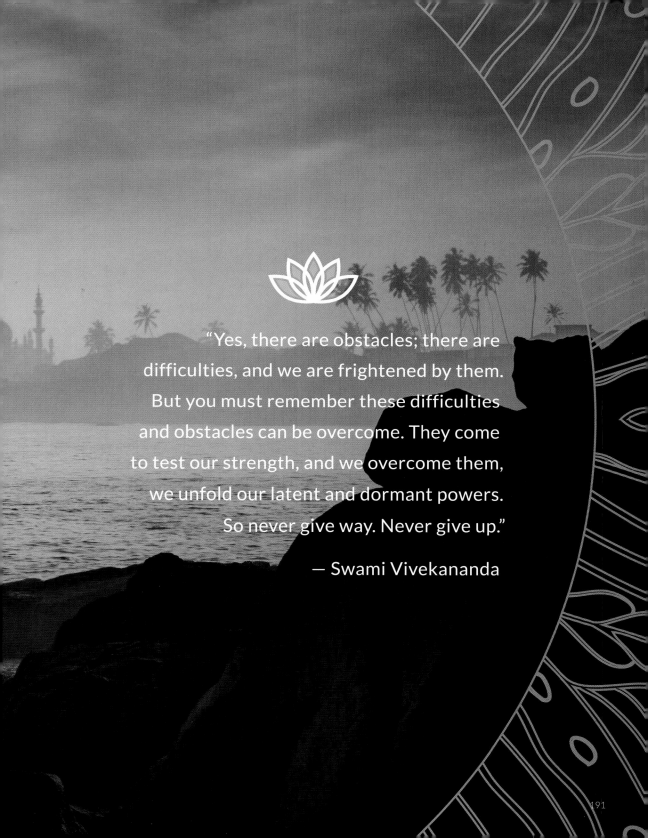

"Yes, there are obstacles; there are difficulties, and we are frightened by them. But you must remember these difficulties and obstacles can be overcome. They come to test our strength, and we overcome them, we unfold our latent and dormant powers. So never give way. Never give up."

— Swami Vivekananda

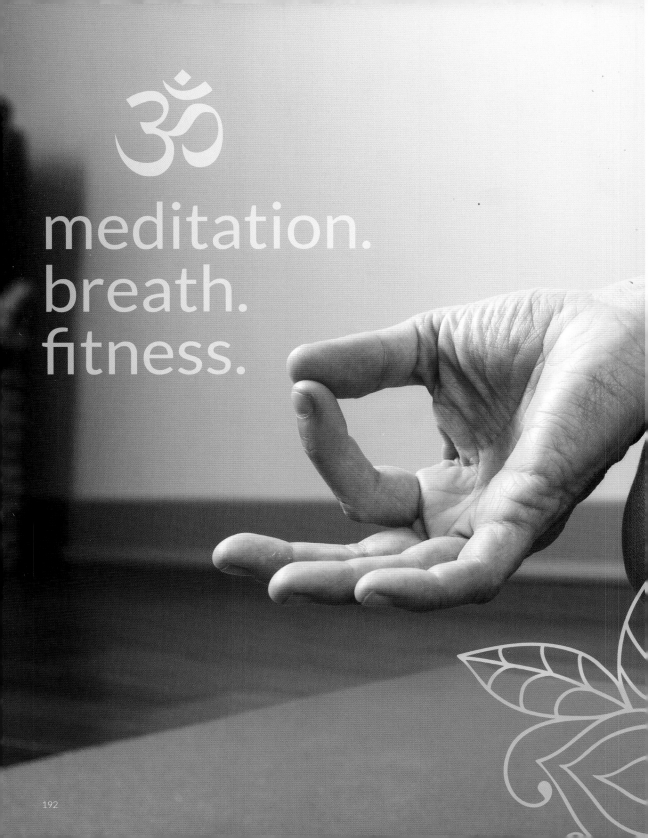

ॐ

meditation.
breath.
fitness.